BODY CARE
JUST FOR
MEN

Natural Health Tips & Herbal Formulas for

- Skin protection
- Sore muscle relief
- Aftershaves, tonics, and more

JIM LONG

STOREY BOOKS

Schoolhouse Road
Pownal, Vermont 05261

*The mission of Storey Communications is to serve our customers
by publishing practical information that encourages personal independence
in harmony with the environment.*

Edited by Deborah Balmuth and Robin Catalano
Cover and text design and production by Mark Tomasi
Cover photograph by © J. A. Nemeth/Picturesque
Photography © Eyewire Images, image styling by Mark Tomasi
Indexed by Nan Badgett, Word•a•bil•i•ty

Storey books are available for special premium and promotional uses and for cus-
tomized editions. For further information, please call Storey's Custom Publishing
Department at 1-800-793-9396.

Printed in the United States by R. R. Donnelley
10 9 8 7 6 5 4 3 2 1

Library of Congress Cataloging-in-Publication Data

Long, Jim, 1946–
    Body care just for men : natural health tips & herbal formulas for skin
    protection, sore muscle relief, aftershaves, tonics, and more / Jim Long.
          p.   cm.
    Includes bibliographical references and index.
    ISBN 1-58017-183-4
    1. Men—Health and hygiene.   2. Beauty, Personal.   3. Herbs—
    Therapeutic use.   I. Title
RA777.8.L66   1999
04234—dc21   99-23381
                                                     CIP

Contents

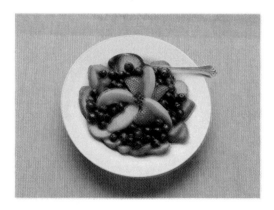

Dedication:
To my mother, Mada Harper Long

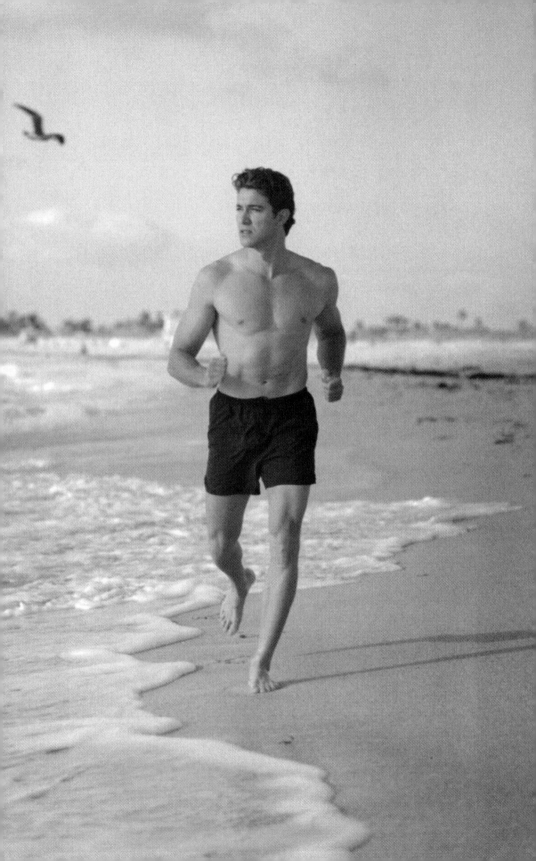

Introduction

caring for yourself naturally

I used to joke with my friends when we were together, trading complaints about growing older when we were all still in our 30s. I'd contend that in my previous life, I had made out the order for my next body: "I remember asking for a superhero's athletic body, 6'2", 185 pounds of lean, mean muscle. Black hair, blue eyes, and tan or dark (not pink) skin. I'd have sharp intelligence, and be surrounded by devoted friends." I'd conclude, "Instead, my hair's falling out, I'm round, not lean, and I'm surrounded by people who whine and complain about growing old. I think my order for this lifetime got lost in the mail."

BEING YOUR BEST

The truth is, no matter what we think we should be like, or want to be like, most of us have to make the best of the hand we are dealt. Few of us can have perfect bodies and look like models. Even the ones whose genetic "roulette wheel" lines up perfectly to give them an outstanding body always wish for a little more, something a little different from what they have. It's human nature to want to be better, to strive and wish for a better hand, a bigger advantage.

Coming to Terms with What You're Given

I remember when I was in my 20s thinking that I simply wouldn't allow myself to age. I would not let my guard down and I would stay young. Older people — out of shape, overweight, bald, wearing glasses, not moving out of the way fast enough — those would never be me. By pure willpower, I would not become them.

The reality is different: different from what I imagined, different from what I believed, and different from what I thought possible. I know men in their 40s who look like they are in their 60s, yet I have known men who were in their 60s and looked 40. While some of the variation comes from how we treat ourselves, it also comes from our genetics — what we were given when we were born.

Regardless of the circumstances, though, most men can do something to improve themselves. Even the 800-pound man who's too big to turn over in bed has an option to quit stuffing food into his mouth. For exercise, he can still move his little finger or wiggle his toes, and that's a start. He can get help, he can improve. So, too, can the man who is at risk for heart disease due to genetic makeup improve his chances of living a longer, better life by changing his diet and habits.

Don't Expect Perfection

I listened to Graham Kerr, a well-known food and health expert and author of an American Heart Association cookbook, as he described his struggle to give guidelines for helping people reduce the amount of fat in their diets. "I became a vegetarian," he said. "I cut out fat, I insisted that my family cut out meat and meat fats. I turned into a radical food monster. Then one day, I caught my son making a bologna sandwich in the kitchen — a food I had forbade even be in the house. We had an ugly fight and it ended in his throwing the bologna in my face," he said. "The funny thing was, not only did the bologna smell good, it made me realize, as the slice fell from my face, that I was trying to make everything be the ideal and it was ruining my relationship with my family."

So Kerr gave up being a strict vegetarian and adopted a more even-handed approach. He decided that worrying about grams of fat in recipes was not the answer to getting busy people to cut down on what kinds of fats they ate. "I came up with a solution that seems more reasonable," he said. "I found that anyone, anywhere, anytime, at home or on the road, can cut out half of the fat in his diet by one simple method: Simply cut it in half. Eat a McDonald's hamburger if that's all you have access to. Don't make a habit of it, but if that's the only choice at that moment, your body still needs food. Simply eat half of the Big Mac and half of the fries, instead of the whole thing. It may not be as healthy as eating something else, but you *can* cut the amount of fat in half by simply eating half."

It makes so much sense to me. If you're in complete control of every meal, if you don't eat out, if you grow all your own food and fix all of your own meals, then eating consistently healthy food is fairly easy. Most people, however, don't live like that. Many have little choice but to eat in a fast-food restaurant part of the time. Most men have stressful, hectic lives. They eat as they drive or work, and not always healthy foods. They're often too tired to exercise and end up gaining weight or losing muscle tone. They groom themselves in a hurry and wind up not liking what they see. But there are ways of improving some areas and of making the best of others. The key, I think, is not to give up on everything just because it isn't all possible. Work on the areas that *are* possible.

Playing Your Hand

My grandfather had that superhero body I always dreamed of. He was 6'2", black-haired, muscular, strong, and athletic. In addition, he worked hard, enjoyed his family, and had the respect of his community. But he died at age 54 from complications of polycystic kidney disease. Even those of us who seem to have it all don't always have the perfect life.

My grandfather had four children, one son and three daughters. All of them had polycystic kidney disease. Out of all of the grandchildren and great-grandchildren (who have been tested), I'm the only one to whom the disease was passed along.

Polycystic kidney disease (PKD for short) is genetic and there's scant treatment save for kidney transplant or dialysis. It's the most common kind of serious kidney disease in Americans, I'm told. No matter how much I wanted to be the "perfect" 6'2", black-haired, strong, athletic man, that's not the hand I was dealt. So do I give up and quit trying to improve my life altogether? No. I walk and exercise regularly. I don't smoke, I drink little alcohol, I don't use salt, I monitor my blood pressure, and I go on with life. I maintain my sense of humor and personal relationships. I work at improving the possibilities for the longest and best life I can have, because it's really the only logical choice.

How Do I Improve My Health?

I've watched men who seemed to be in much better health than I let themselves go to pieces. They chain smoke, they don't get enough rest, they sit around feeling sorry that they didn't turn out the way they thought they would. There's *always* something a man can do to improve his life. It might be as simple as not eating the other half of the Big Mac, or it might be cutting out cigarettes and getting some exercise. Here are the top five practices that I believe are important for a man in maintaining his health.

Step 1: Be Happy

This is important for your health. If you wait until you *are* happy, you'll never *be* happy. It's not a place you arrive at one day and say, " This is it. This is pure happiness, this is what I've been waiting for all my life." There's a choice every day. You can get up cussing at the world and whining that life's got the best of you and nothing is right, or you can get up and decide, "I'm going to be happy today." Happiness is a state of mind, not a place and not a date on a calendar. And happiness is a process, something to enjoy along the way.

My grandmother told me when I was in my 20s that I had a choice between working all my life at a thankless job, much like my parents, or, instead, doing what I really loved. It was a hard lesson for me and it

→ **Educate Yourself about Kidney Disease**

Approximately 1.2 million men suffer from various kinds of kidney disease. If you want to know more about dialysis, transplants, or referral to specific kidney foundations for yourself or a family member, call the American Association of Kidney Patients (see Resources).

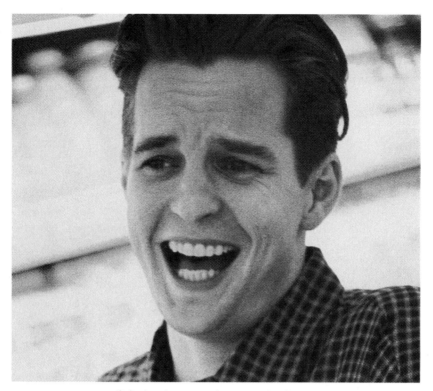

Learn to enjoy yourself; feeling happy and contented is the most important step for a healthy life.

took over 20 years for her words to finally soak in. "You have a choice," she said. "Live your life doing what everyone else expects you to do, or gather up the courage to do what *you* most want to do." There are probably the same number of days in a lifetime whether you spend them being miserable, doing what's expected of you regardless of whether or not it makes you happy, or whether you do what gives you joy and pleasure.

Working at something that makes you happy will affect every other part of your existence. I run an herb business, making herbal products, working at home with my catalog business. Some days, when I'm harvesting herbs from my garden, bundling them and getting them ready to dry in the drying room, I actually get silly and laugh right out loud. The goats and geese in the barnyard may look up at the sound of my voice. I've actually yelled out to them, "Can you believe it? This is fun, this is what I've always wanted to do. And best of all, it's my job. It's what I'm paid to do!" So, being happy is at the top of the list of things I think a man can, and should, do for himself. If he's miserable at what he does in life, every other part of his life will suffer — whether it's his relationships, spirit, business, or health. As my grandmother said, "Do what you really love first and everything else will fall into place."

Step 2: Improve Your Health

If you're a muscle-bound stud with every part of your body buffed and polished, go work on something else. But if you're an average Joe, there's always something you can do to improve your physical health. Eat half of the Big Mac instead of the whole thing. Even better, eat a big salad that's full of a variety of vegetables and fruit. If you're a serious vegetarian, listen to your body's cravings; those cravings will tell you if you aren't getting all the protein and nutrients you need for a healthy body. If you find that you're craving meat, it might be that you need to look into dairy or other protein sources. The key, I think, is to listen to your body and give it the good, healthy food it needs to keep running smoothly. Listen to the cravings and learn from them, but don't let them rule your life.

The point is, we all have to start with the body and health we've received. We can't go back and change our genes and we can't help the food binge we went on three days ago. The one thing we *can* do is have control over what we eat today. Make sure it's better for you than what you ate yesterday. Try a bit more exercise than before. Get naked, stand in front of a full-length mirror, and say, "Well, you're all I've got. Now, how can I make this body a little better?"

Step 3: Forgive Yourself for Your Imperfections

I used to hate my body when I was growing up. I always wanted slim hips and wide shoulders and longer legs. In fourth grade I would hang upside down on the playground equipment, hoping that with enough hanging, gravity would lengthen my legs and I could run faster. In my early teens, I was so frustrated that my body wasn't what I wanted it to be that I'd stand in a doorway and pull the door closed hard against my hips, hoping that with enough pressure I could mash them into a narrower shape.

Most men would like their bodies to be better. Even the "perfect bodies" that athletes and models have are never quite enough. If you ask one of those guys, "Are you completely happy with your body?" the really honest answer is always something like, "I'd really like my nose to be different" or "My muscle definition could be better." Every man's body is different and that difference is what makes us interesting. Forgive yourself for having fat ankles, wide hips, or whatever it is that you think makes you less worthy. Laugh at yourself, have fun with yourself, but, most of all, forgive yourself for not being perfect and get on with being the best *imperfect* guy you can be.

Step 4: Do *Something*

I used to know a guy whose watchword for each day was, "Well, let's do something, even if it's wrong." I always admired that; it meant that he was going to take action based on his best judgment, even if it turned out later to be wrong.

I know men who are very talented, maybe at sports, or at art or electronics, but they spend their time afraid to try, instead wishing they had success with these occupations. They bemoan the fact that they haven't gotten anywhere in life. I think the only difference between achieving success and suffering failure is that some people try and others don't. No matter how good you may be at mechanics, cartooning, design, or architecture, you'll never get anywhere unless you get off that couch and try. Failing at something is nothing to be embarrassed about. Not trying in the first place is a great shame.

Step 5: Never Stop

Part of giving up may have to do with genetics or a person's emotional makeup. But the other part is simply a decision. My father, who was never a very happy person, gave up on life when he retired. He spent the next 20 years sitting in his recliner, lamenting the fact that something was always wrong. "If it's not the water heater or hemmorhoids or the roof, it's something else," he'd say.

By contrast, I watched my mother struggle with cancer over a 10-year period. She loved life and was interested in just about everything around her. Even in her last months, knowing that she was near death, she continued to read, to learn, to teach herself new ways of doing things. She decided every day that life was worth one more effort. She stayed involved, she stayed connected to people around her, and she never gave up.

Life can be a burden, a misery to be endured, or you can decide that you'll make the most of what's available and engage in it yourself. My theory is that life is actually a kind of grade-school class. We learn our lessons as we go along and we're graded not on whether we succeed or fail, but on how well we study.

Herbal Tips to Keep the Human "Vehicle" Running Better

If you've never made anything from herbs, you may feel intimidated at not knowing where to start. Well, good news, fella! Equipment and supplies are simple. You'll need to look through the glossary, which answers questions about where to look for unusual products (gum resins, oils, and so on). In the Resources section are my recommendations for places that will sell you those items if you don't have ready access to them.

Getting Started

When it comes to herbs, I encourage you to grow your own. Because herbs are small in size, relatively speaking (unlike shrubbery in the landscape, for instance), and because you harvest the same plant repeatedly, you can grow a dozen or more plants in a 2-foot by 10-foot space. Or you can grow herbs in patio pots, even in a windowsill planter if you live in an apartment. I recommend my own book, *Herbs, Just for Fun,* as a simple beginner's guide. For a larger tome, Betty Jacobs's *Growing & Using Herbs Successfully* (Storey Books, 1981) is a good bet. Herbs are simple and forgiving, yet will yield powerful uses.

But if you don't choose to grow your own herbs, pick one or more of the sources in this book for dried herbs. They offer their products by mail and most sell in small amounts. Or look in your local health-food store or herb shop, as many sell herbs in bulk.

Collecting Materials and Equipment

Making your own herbal preparations is both fun and rewarding. As you gain knowledge about how to use herbs and how they work, you will soon be concocting your own recipes. By making your own preparations, you are participating in improving your health, rather than relying on manufacturers to do it for you.

Here are some basic preparation and storage items that are good to keep on hand:

Food processor and microwave oven. For making salves, tinctures, or oils, it's nice, but not absolutely necessary, to have a food processor and a microwave. Obviously, because some of these formulas were used before or during the Civil War, there were no food processors or microwaves then; you can certainly work without them.

Double boiler. Some of the instructions in the following chapters call for melting beeswax in the microwave. You can also melt it in a double boiler (not in a pan directly over a hot burner, however, as beeswax catches fire easily). Another method that works well is to put a skillet upside down on the stove burner. Place a small pan atop that and slowly melt the wax that way. However, a microwave works best, in my opinion.

Product containers. Other items that you might want to have on hand are a few glass or plastic bottles for oils and shaker containers for foot powders. There are companies that will sell you one, two, or more of these items. Or you can save a few empty bottles and salve containers, wash them out, and keep them for making your own products. Glass is usually recommended, but plastic containers can be used if that's all you have. Plastic sometimes absorbs smells that can be difficult to wash out.

Saucepans and herb containers. The only other pieces of equipment you'll need are a small pan or two for heating oil and some containers, like plastic freezer containers or plastic zipper-lock bags, for storing dried herbs and powders. Although it's not a necessity, I often use a blender when the dried herbs are not completely powdered. I'll whir up the dry herbs in the blender — removing any stems that don't get ground — before putting them in a salve.

Vodka. For making tinctures, I usually use the cheapest vodka I can find. Vodka works as well as brandy. If you buy it on sale, you can have it on hand when you are ready to make something.

A Few Cautions

Although herbs are all-natural ingredients, they and their products still need to be purchased, used, and stored with care. Here are some issues to keep in mind when preparing and using herbal formulas.

Fresh or Dried?

Why fresh *or* dried herbs in some of the recipes you'll find in this book? Dried herbs are more concentrated because the moisture has been removed. Cookbook and many body-care recipes generally call for twice as much fresh herb as dried.

However, I've found that the strength of dried herbs varies a great deal. A dried herb loses half of its flavor after about nine months. As it may have already been in a warehouse for six months, on the grocery store shelf for three months, and in your kitchen for six months, it could easily be one or two years since the herb was freshly picked where it was grown. Therefore, I simply use the same measurement for fresh or dried herbs in these recipes. Fresh is always better, but dried herbs will do.

Grinding Herbs

Some people will try to convince you that in order to grind up herbs you must only use a mortar and pestle or a special (expensive) spice grinder. As my Brit friends say, "Poppycock!" If the herbalists of the previous century had good blenders they would never have spent hours pounding and grinding. A blender works great for turning bulk herbs into ground herbs or powder. It's great for mixing oils and herbs, as well.

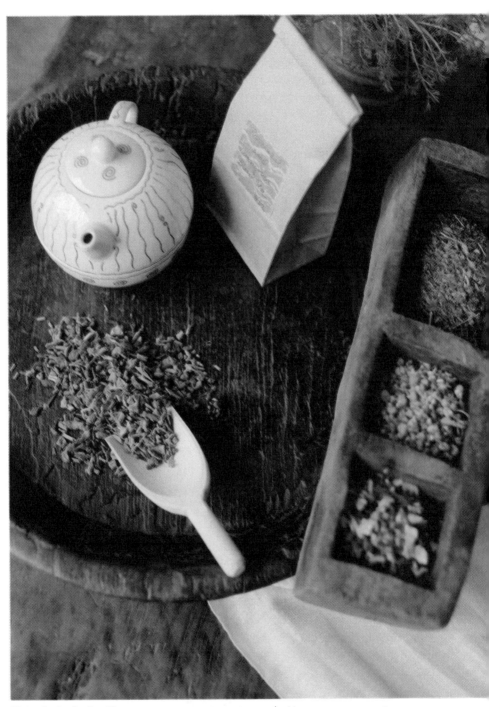

Using herbs for health care is not as exotic as it sounds. You can use a great variety of herbs in many simple personal-care formulas.

You won't want to grind up herbs you aren't going to use immediately, as ground herbs lose their strength faster than herbs that are left in bigger pieces. But for making the herbal preparations found in this book, a blender works very well.

Drying Herbs

Do not use a microwave to dry herbs. While it is fast, it destroys the essential oils of the plant, leaving you with a useless pile of plant material. If you don't believe me, put a few fresh herbs in the microwave and dry them. Notice that when you open the door, you get a strong odor of herbs in the air. That's the vapor of the oils that should have stayed in the plant material, the very oils that make these formulas effective.

So what's the best way to dry them for use in these recipes? Pick a handful of fresh herbs and place them in a plain paper (not plastic) bag, close it by folding it over, and place the bag on the dashboard of your car. One day on the dash will usually dry herbs; don't leave them out for more than two days. Any longer, and the sunlight will begin to break down the essential oils in the herbs.

Another method, good for larger amounts of herbs, is to place them in paper grocery bags, three or four handfuls of herbs per bag, and partially close the bags. Place those in the trunk of your car. Check them daily, stir the herbs a bit, and as soon as the herbs are crisp — that is, when the leaves and stems snap when bent — remove them and store in airtight containers away from light. In summer, the herbs will dry in about two to four days.

About Essential Oils

Essential oils are the fragrant oils of a plant. To obtain the oil, plants are harvested in large quantities, the plants or flowers are crushed to break up the oil cells, then the oil is extracted by steam distillation. It may take hundreds of pounds, or more, of a particular flower to yield a few ounces of oil. That process, and the material and labor required, is what makes an oil, such as attar of rose oil, so expensive (hundreds of dollars an ounce).

Fragrance oils, which should not be used for most body-care recipes, are simply chemical concoctions made to smell like a particular fragrance. Don't substitute — they're not the same thing! Essential oils should never be applied directly to the skin; the exception is lavender oil, which is sometimes applied to the fingertips and rubbed into the temples for headache. All other oils should be diluted before application.

Using Plastic Wrap and Containers

Some researchers believe that certain kinds of plastic wrap release toxins when heated. Be sure that your plastic wrap is approved for microwave use (not all wraps are) before heating. This will help guard you against potential contaminants.

Likewise, many herbalists prefer glass over plastic storage containers, since the volatile oils in herbs may react with the plastic. If you have a glass container use it, but if not plastic works just as well, in my opinion. The key is to store dried herbs in airtight containers or bags, in a dark place. Light breaks down the color of herbs, which is an indication that the essential oils are leaving the plant and, thus, the flavor and useful parts as well.

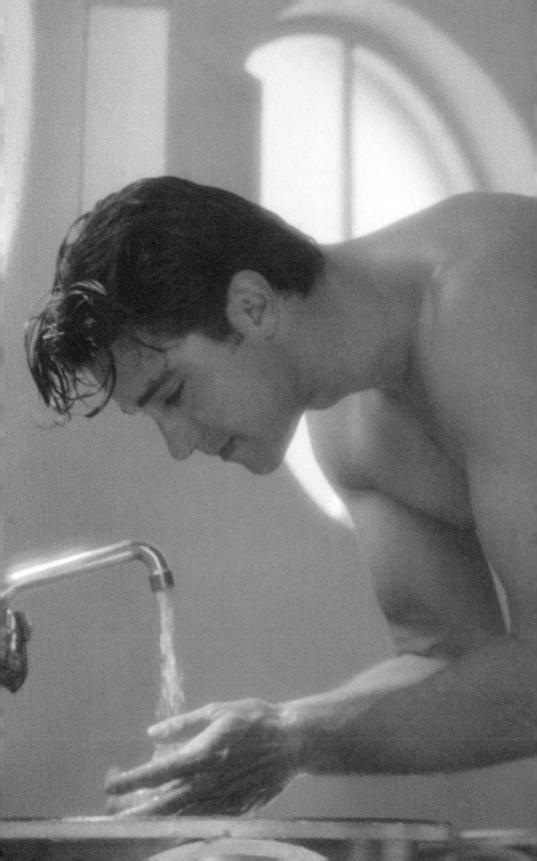

Chapter 1

guidelines for overall health

I've seen men who smoked heavily, drank excessively, seldom slept the night through, ate greasy fast food full-time, then were surprised when they had a massive heart attack or cancer. If we expect to have good health, we have to see that health as a cumulative effort. It sounds like a page out of our general health book back in high school, but getting enough sleep and rest, eating a healthy diet, being happy, having faith in something, and having people around you who love and care for you are all important for living the best, longest, and healthiest life you can. Take care of your body and chances are it won't let you down.

THE EFFECTS OF DIET ON HEALTH

We have known for generations how we *should* eat for our maximum health, even if most men choose not to. I hold up, as an example of our knowing, the 1828 book called *The Indian Physician*, by Dr. Jonas Rishel (the actual title is *The Indian Physician — Containing a New System of Practice Founded on Medical Plants Together with a Description of Their Properties, Localities, and Methods of Using and Preparing Them; A Treatise on the Causes and Symptoms of Disease, Which Are Incident to Human Nature, with a Safe and Sovereign Cure for Them and the Mode of Treatment, in Any Stage of Disease, for the*

Use of Families and Practitioners of Medicine). It was published at a time when there was a great need for everyday health material, little information was available, and long book titles were in vogue.

Dr. Rishel was born in 1788 and lived and practiced medicine first in eastern Pennsylvania, moving later to the frontier area of Ohio, the same basic route that my own family took when going west. The Long family arrived in America about 1647 and lived first in Virginia, then in Pennsylvania, and moved to Ohio and on to Indiana, Iowa, Kansas, and Missouri. I can't prove it, but I'd like to believe that the Longs knew Dr. Rishel's book. His was just about the only family medical book available in that area, and it is said that he was widely respected for his commonsense approach to medicine — including his nonacceptance of the practice of "bleeding," which often proved fatal and didn't fall out of fashion until nearly the time of the Civil War.

Here is what Rishel said in 1828 about diet, on the page entitled "Diet of Manhood": "A diet of young meat, with fruits and fresh vegetables has been recommended . . . also the use of wine diluted with water. Temperance, both with respect to food and drink, cannot be too scrupulously observed, by persons of every age." In some cases he recommended a vegetarian diet, but always he urged a well-balanced, moderate diet.

Dr. Rishel's book gives descriptions of many plants still in use today (along with a number that are not). His salves, tinctures, and syrups were everyday remedies for many families.

Improve Your Diet

We have a schedule — certain work we must do each day, obligations, activities, worry. Many of us don't feel that we can just simply change our lifestyle into one that's healthy. But I suggest that we all work on areas on which we can have some effect. Maybe it's as simple as drinking juice instead of soda part of the time. Maybe it's merely leaving out two cigarettes a day, or eating half the french fries instead of the whole bag.

Lots of us read the dessert menu and say to ourselves, "Eating that piece of banana cream pie doesn't make one bit of difference." But over time, all of those pieces of banana cream pie *do* make a difference. Instead of looking at those activities as if you are giving up something, take the attitude that you are making a contribution. Eat something healthy at every opportunity. Make a rule for yourself: Decide that every meal should include at least one fresh vegetable or fruit. Let's hope it's more than the lettuce on a Burger King Whopper, of course, but forgive yourself if it isn't and try to do better at the next meal.

Keep your bowels regular, eat roughage, make sure you get five servings of fruits and vegetables every day — these go a long way toward keeping your body working as it was designed to. Cut out the fat, replace the french fries with a celery stick, drink cranberry-raspberry or orange juice instead of a Coke, and you've made a deposit on your health. Do it often and it becomes a healthy habit.

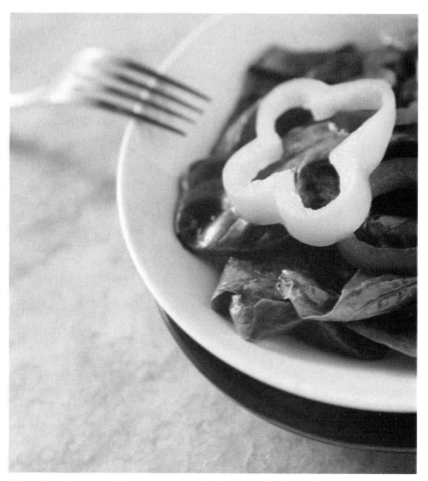

A healthy diet goes a long way toward making you feel good. Incorporate a variety of fruits and vegetables in your diet for best effect.

Actually Edible Oatmeal

We know that oatmeal is good for us. Two cups contain about 50 grams of carbohydrates, giving slow-release and long-burning energy. Those two cups also provide 8 grams of fiber, with only 5 grams of fat, but most oatmeal is about as tasty as wallpaper paste. Here's a recipe to make the oatmeal even more energy-efficient and really good-tasting, as well.

> 2 tablespoons raisins
> 1 apple, finely chopped
> 1½ cups apple juice
> ¾ cup dry quick oats
> Pinch of cinnamon
> Dark honey or maple syrup (optional)

Combine the raisins, chopped apple, and apple juice in a microwave-proof bowl. Cover with plastic wrap and heat on high in the microwave for 1 minute, or until the liquid begins to bubble on the edges. Add the oats and cinnamon and stir, then microwave until thickened, about another 30 seconds. Sweeten with the dark honey or maple syrup, if desired (the apple juice and raisins make it somewhat sweet already).

→ Healthy Honey?

Dark, thick honey has been shown to be high in antioxidants. Researchers at the University of Illinois tested 14 varieties of honey and found that darker honey, such as that from buckwheat, sunflower, and Christmasberry, is higher in antioxidants and contains vitamins C and E, along with beta-carotene. "By using honey exclusively instead of sugar," says researcher May Berenbaum, Ph.D., "you can significantly increase your intake of antioxidants." You may recall that antioxidants are believed to help prevent the cell damage that can lead to heart disease and some kinds of cancer.

Power Take-Off (PTO) Oatmeal

The PTO connector is where the power is transferred from a motor to equipment, as in tractors and heavy machinery. This breakfast oatmeal packs plenty of power to keep you full of energy until lunchtime. The fruit adds a sweet taste, nice flavor, and vitamins. With toast and juice, this is a low-calorie, low-fat, quick breakfast.

1 cup water
1/4 cup raisins
3 to 4 dried apricots, cut up
2 tablespoons dried cranberries
1/2 cup quick oatmeal
1/2 cup skim or 1% milk (optional)

Heat the water in a saucepan. Add the raisins, apricots, and cranberries, and let simmer for about 1 minute. Add the oatmeal and stir, simmering for another minute. Cover the pan and remove from the heat. Serve the oatmeal with the skim or 1% milk, if desired, accompanied by toast and juice.

Gas Pain Tea

No matter how much healthy stuff a guy eats, he'll still have occasional gas pains. Maybe it's a poor food combination, maybe it's just the way our bodies are built. Here's an apothecary's gas pain remedy that works well. Use dried herbs for best effect.

1/2 cup peppermint leaves
1/4 cup chamomile flowers
2 tablespoons lemon balm leaves
1 tablespoon anise seed
1 tablespoon fennel seed
1 tablespoon lavender flowers

1. Mix together all ingredients and store in an airtight container away from direct light.
2. Put 2 teaspoons of the mix into a tea infuser or tea strainer in a large cup. Pour 1 cup of boiling water over the herbs, and let steep, covered, for 5 to 7 minutes. Strain out the herbs, and drink.

Decrease Your Chances for Broken Bones

Forrest Nielson, Ph.D., who led a study for the USDA, says, "Drinking large amounts of fructose changes how your body metabolizes the minerals responsible for healthy bones." The study called for 11 men to drink five cans of cola daily for three months. After the three months, the men had lost about 10 percent more phosphorus through their urine than normal, and had also absorbed less calcium. Dr. Nielsen stresses that drinking more than two cans of soda per day could lead to deterioration of bones.

Eating a healthy diet and getting sufficient calcium (especially through dairy products and leafy green vegetables), exercise, and rest will all contribute to healthy, strong bones.

Reduce Your Risk of Cancer

A good diet is the best cancer preventive we have. Vegetables rich in beta-carotene and other antioxidants are the most important foods you can add to your menu. Leafy dark green vegetables, in particular, are loaded with antioxidants.

Broccoli contains concentrations of sulforaphane, an anticancer compound. To get the sufficient amount to help decrease your chances of colon cancer, you'd have to eat about 2 pounds of broccoli per week. I think that would be impossible for most men to tolerate. However, a study published in the *Proceedings of the National Academy of Sciences* says that broccoli sprouts contain up to 50 times more anticancer chemical as the mature vegetable.

Broccoli sprouts look much like alfalfa or radish sprouts, but with much better flavor. "Because of the high content of sulforaphane, it's possible to consume far smaller quantities of the sprouts and get the same protection," Dr. Paul Talalay, head of research at Johns Hopkins University, says.

Healthy Snacking

I like cookies, most any kind of cookies — except for chocolate chip, which I had to learn to like. For 10 years, my ex-wife made only one kind of cookie; she made chocolate-chip cookies, even though she knew I didn't care for them. The smell of freshly baking cookies is a sweet smell to any man, and over time I gave in and acquired a taste for them. Since being single, I've learned to make really good chocolate-chip cookies and realized that it wasn't the cookies, it was my wife's lousy recipe.

Cookies are fine as a treat, but don't snack on them too often; there are lots of other alternatives that are much healthier. Some examples of healthy snacks for men are fresh fruits, green and yellow raw vegetables, grains, pumpkin seeds, almonds, whole wheat breads, whole grain cereals, sprouts, low-fat yogurt, and fruit and vegetable juices (especially fresh).

Man-Snacks (Manpower Cookies)

I like to carry these cookies in my pocket when I go hiking along the lakeshore, or when I take the tackle box, rod, and reel and pretend to catch fish. Teens enjoy these cookies; just don't tell them that they're healthy or they'll probably quit liking them.

This recipe makes about 30 two-inch, chewy energy cookies.

> ½ pound (2 sticks) butter or margarine,
>   softened in microwave
> 1 cup brown sugar, packed tight
> 2 eggs
> 1 teaspoon vanilla
> 1 good pinch of cinnamon
> 2 cups all-purpose flour
> 2 cups oats (quick-cooking or regular)
> 1 teaspoon baking soda
> 1 teaspoon baking powder
> ½ cup any kind of raisins
> ½ cup dried apricots or dried pineapple (optional)
> ½ cup nuts (walnuts, pecans, peanuts, sunflower
>   seeds, or a combination; optional)
> ½ cup dry cereal, any kind works (optional)

1. Preheat oven to 350°F. In a large mixing bowl, combine the butter and brown sugar, mixing briefly. Stir in the eggs, vanilla, and cinnamon.
2. Add the flour, oats, baking soda, baking powder, and raisins. This makes a very stiff batter; use a large wooden spoon or your hands to stir (hands work better). Add any of the optional ingredients, if desired. Add another egg if needed to stiffen, and mix again.
3. Drop batter onto a cookie sheet by tablespoonful, about an inch apart. Bake for 8 to 10 minutes. Remove with a spatula and let cool in single layers on plates.

How to Cut Back Safely

Not long ago I was interviewing some sports people about their own special remedies. I talked with a guy in a gym as he worked out about how he maintained his health. He told me he felt like he was gaining weight and so was on a fast, plus giving extra attention to his midsection. He looked fit, so I was curious about his fasting regimen. As he worked out, I asked him, "What kind of fast are you on?"

I was startled at the guy's answer: "Pepsi," he said. "I haven't eaten any food or drunk anything except Diet Pepsi for the past 12 days." He worked nights as a stripper in clubs that cater to women, and did modeling jobs for magazines the rest of the time. I know enough about nutrition to know that although he now looked fit and trim, treating his body this way for very long would do some awful things to his overall health, and no amount of Diet Pepsi and workouts would give him back his health.

But there are some safe ways to fast, if you really need to cut back on calories and fat. A pharmacist friend of mine always recommended a watermelon fast for people who wanted to cleanse their body or lose weight. "The juice from watermelon contains enough nutrients that you don't crave food as much as you do on a straight water fast," he'd said. "Watermelon stops the craving and you're not as weak, either." If you choose the watermelon fast, simply juice a watermelon, removing the seeds and pulp, and drink 4 to 6 glasses of the juice daily, with lots of water in between. Fasting isn't for everyone, though. Always ask your doctor or healthcare provider before starting on a fast.

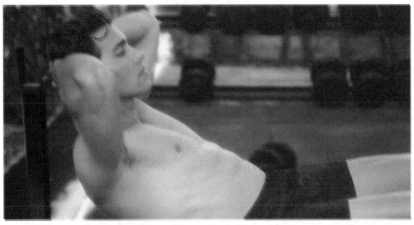

Exercise is a great way to lose weight and enhance muscle tone. But don't overdo it, especially if you are also fasting.

Reducing & Fasting Tea

I've known quite a number of people who've used this with success, but check with a qualified healthcare provider first. The Reducing & Fasting Tea can be used by itself or as part of the watermelon juice fast.

> 1 ounce licorice powder (see box)
> 2 ounces dandelion leaves
> 2 ounces fennel seed
> 4 ounces chickweed
> 2 ounces kelp

1. Mix all ingredients and store in an airtight container. Store in a cool, dark place.

2. To use, in a medium saucepan bring 1½ gallons of water to a boil and add the herb mix. Simmer, covered, for about 1 minute, then remove from the heat and let steep for an hour. Strain out the herbs and discard. Keep the liquid in the refrigerator. The pharmacist's instructions recommend drinking 1 cup of this warmed liquid three times a day, with glasses of water or juice in between.

A Warning on Licorice

Licorice shouldn't be used by people who are on blood pressure–lowering medications, according to 7Song, an herbal practitioner in Ithaca, New York. Licorice can cause salt and water retention, he said. Steven Foster, in *The Encyclopedia of Natural Ingredients Used in Food, Drugs, and Cosmetics*, says that licorice is known to "exhibit . . . sodium retention and potassium loss leading to hypertension." If you are prone to hypertension or sodium retention, leave the licorice out of this formula.

Get Lots of Sleep

It's estimated that more than 10 million people regularly rely on pills to get enough sleep. Insomnia can be caused by job stress, worry, fear, fatigue, and many other factors. If it's a persistent problem, see a doctor or counselor. But if sleeplessness isn't common for you, you can likely find a simple remedy.

A relaxing bath before bedtime — in a tub, not a shower — can be soothing. Of course, there's not much that puts a man to sleep faster than a good round of sex. For lots of men, the physical release brings on sleep, like they've taken a hammer to the back of the head.

For men who don't exercise enough during the day, exercise in the early evening can be beneficial. You don't want to do the exercise right before bedtime, of course, as you'll be raising your metabolism and blood pressure at a time when it should be slowing down. But exercising after work or before dinner, eating a light meal, then relaxing in your favorite chair with a good book and a soothing beverage is a good plan. Men who don't exercise, bring work home, gulp or skip their dinner, down several mixed drinks, worry about the following day, work until midnight, and then expect to lie down and drop off to sleep are candidates for long-term insomnia.

If you fall into that category, my suggestion is that you take a long, hard look at the work you do. What earthly reason, what possible excuse, can there be to have a job that is so stressful and demanding that you can't use part of the evening to relax and rejuvenate yourself for the following day? If you treated your car as you are treating yourself, it would be stalled on the freeway.

→ Sleep Tip

When you get up during the night for a trip to the bathroom, you'll have an easier time going back to sleep if you don't turn on the lights. Use low-watt, cool blue LED night lights around the house so that turning on lamps isn't necessary. Exposure to bright light in the night causes your body to produce melatonin, a hormone that regulates sleeping and waking cycles. Interrupting the cycle makes it harder to go back to sleep.

Use Herbs to Treat Insomnia

Several herbs are helpful for sleep for the average guy with occasional sleeplessness. These are:

- Lemon balm *(Melissa officinalis)*
- Valerian *(Valeriana officinalis)*
- Passionflower *(Passiflora incarnata)*
- Chamomile *(Matricaria recutita)*
- Catnip *(Nepeta cataria)*
- Hops *(Humulus lupulus)*

Each of these herbs will work by itself. A cup of chamomile tea before bedtime is soothing and relaxing. So is catnip tea (it is soothing to humans; however, cats have quite a different reaction).

Valerian, an herb that is approved by Commission E, the body of scientists that advises the German government about herb use, considers valerian so safe that it even recommends drinking the herb in tea throughout the day to relieve anxiety and nervousness. A cup of valerian tea 30 minutes before bedtime is relaxing and encourages sleep for many people, although a very small percentage of people will have the opposite reaction. However, this herb just plain stinks. Unless you're used to the smell, you might prefer to take this herb in capsule or tincture form instead of tea.

Nature's Herbs brand valerian combination, available in 390 mg capsules, contains valerian, hops, wood betony, skullcap, black cohosh, and passionflower and is easy to carry along when you travel. I keep a few capsules in my shaving kit when I go on lecture trips. If I'm having trouble sleeping, I take three capsules before bedtime. Avoid carbonated beverages and anything with sugar right before you go to sleep. Sugar promotes energy and activity, which fight against sleep.

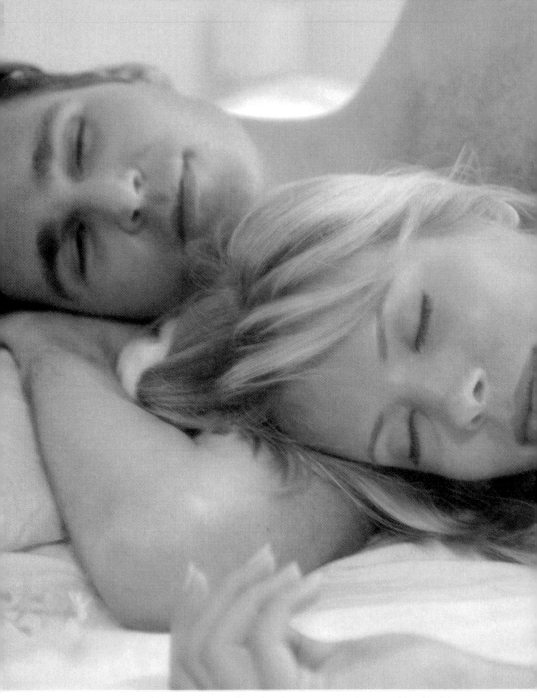

Getting an adequate amount of quality sleep is essential to good health. Most men need between seven and nine hours of sleep per night.

Sleepy Tea

Here's a tea that combines the best of the sleep-inducing herbs. Unlike sleep-ing pills, which have side effects, there is no chemical hangover and no chance of overdose from using these herbs. All herbs used in this formula are dried.

Note: *If you have an allergy to ragweed, leave chamomile out of this mix. A very few people who are allergic to ragweed sometimes show some reaction to chamomile.*

> 1 cup lemon balm leaves
> 1 cup passionflower leaves
> ½ cup chamomile
> ½ cup catnip
> ½ cup hops
> ½ cup lavender flowers
> ½ cup dried orange peel

1. Mix all ingredients and store in an airtight container or bag. Store in a cool, dark place.

2. To use, put 2 heaping teaspoons of the mixture in a tea infuser (tea ball) and place in a large cup. Pour 1 cup of boiling water over the mixture and let steep, covered, for 7 minutes. Drink while still warm, 30 minutes before bedtime. Try the tea every night for a while for best effect.

Restful Sleep Pillow

Certain herbs have been found to encourage sleep. This recipe has helped ease the nightmares of several Vietnam War veterans; I've received wonderful thank-you letters from them praising this blend. If you want to read more about this topic, see my book Making Herbal Dream Pillows *from Storey Books.*

> 2 tablespoons lavender flowers
> 2 tablespoons mugwort
> 2 tablespoons sweet hops

Mix the herbs and put them into a 3 x 5-inch cotton drawstring bag or an old sock. Tie closed. Place the little bag in your pillowcase; the key is to get the herb blend near your nose as you sleep.

Monitoring Your Health

There are always clues to good or bad health. A deep vertical crease down the middle of your earlobe is a fairly reliable sign of certain kinds of heart disease, claim researchers for *Men's Health* magazine. Sudden changes in skin color, eyelids that start to droop, frequent cold sores, eyes that burn or itch, are all signs of changes in health. Listen to your body. If you feel bad more often than you feel good, please consult a healthcare professional.

Accessing Information

You might want to check out Gene Weingarten's enlightening book *The Hypochondriac's Guide to Life. And Death.,* in which you can research specific symptoms and their causes. A lifetime hypochondriac himself, Weingarten offers a kind of rundown of symptoms, a checkup list, if you will, like an encyclopedia of what to worry about and what not to worry about, as a guide for when to see a doctor.

For information about gastrointestinal problems, you can call the toll-free number of the International Foundation for Functional Gastrointestinal Disorders (IFFGD) Monday through Friday, for remedies, referrals, and information about constipation, diarrhea, and irritable-bowel syndrome. If you want information about combining medicines, go to the Johns Hopkins Health Information Web site, which lists interactions, proper usages, and side effects of thousands of drugs. You can search by brand name or generic name or simply browse the index.

An excellent source for up-to-date health information, including mainstream, alternative, and herbal medicines and their effectiveness,

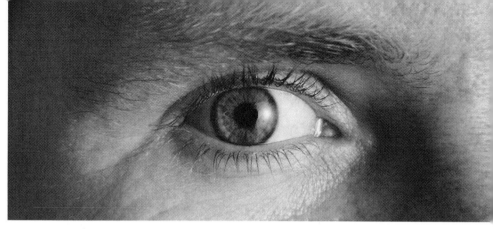

Expect to see changes in your body as you age. While most changes are a normal part of the process, you should seek the advice of a healthcare professional for any alterations that cause pain or discomfort.

is the Web site of the People's Pharmacy show, aired on Public Radio stations across the nation. And for questions about diabetes and the various means of controlling that disease, contact the American Diabetes Association. See Resources for phone numbers or Internet addresses of all of these organizations.

Dealing with Changes

As everyone knows, the body changes over time. We adapt to most changes without even thinking about them, but sometimes a change can be troublesome. Skin and nails can be affected by climate, diet, the body's overall health, and even medications. If persistent or severe problems occur, see a dermatologist or healthcare provider. For some of the minor complaints, here are a few easy herbal formulas.

Skin

Moving from one part of the country to another for a job can have an effect on the oiliness of the skin, says Nancy Silverburg, M.D., an assistant clinical professor of dermatology at the University of California at Irvine: "Climate changes like this can have a big impact on your skin conditions." If oiliness is a problem after moving to a new location (and it hasn't been in the past), she recommends washing the face with mild soap and water three or four times a day. If the condition persists or is severe, she recommends Seban, an over-the-counter product that removes oil from the skin and keeps it from returning for several hours.

Myrrh and Goldenseal Salve

My pharmacist friend Jerry Stamps made this formula as an ointment, but I prefer the more solid salve; if you prefer a liquid form, leave out the beeswax. This soothes insect bites and helps speed up healing of wounds, nicks, scratches, and scrapes anywhere on the body, even little cuts from shaving.

If a double boiler isn't handy, put the same ingredients in a slow cooker, on the lowest setting, and leave it for a couple of hours. Add the lavender oil just before pouring.

¼ cup coconut oil
¼ cup mineral oil
2 ounces petroleum jelly
1 tablespoon powdered organically grown goldenseal root
1 ounce comfrey leaves, finely ground
1 tablespoon powdered myrrh
2 heaping tablespoons beeswax shavings
10 drops lavender essential oil

1. Heat the coconut oil, mineral oil, and petroleum jelly in a double boiler or slow cooker. Add the goldenseal, comfrey, and myrrh, and keep it very warm, but not boiling, for about 1 hour. Remove from the heat and let cool overnight.

2. Reheat the liquid. Add the beeswax shavings and stir until they are completely dissolved. Remove from heat and add the lavender oil, stir again, and pour into a salve container or small bowl. Allow to set, covered, until cool and semi-firm. Some of the herb sediment will settle at the bottom, but don't be concerned.

3. Use as you would any salve on small injuries, bites, and scratches.

Fingernails

Relocations, medication, climate, weather changes, and body changes can have an effect on the nails. Sometimes, for no apparent reason, the fingernails start to get brittle. Frequent soaks in a hot tub can even cause nails to become brittle. Excessive brittleness can be a sign of medical problems, and if the condition persists, check with your doctor. But occasional nail brittleness isn't uncommon. A good daily multivitamin and a well-balanced diet are good preventives.

Fingernail Hardener

Here's a formula from my pharmacist friend Jerry for hardening the nails.

3 tablespoons water
1 tablespoon glycerin
1 teaspoon powdered alum

1. Mix all ingredients well. Store in an airtight container.
2. To use, before bedtime wipe the mixture on your nails with a small brush. Remove in the morning with rubbing alcohol on a cotton ball or cloth. Use a moisturizing hand lotion, massaging in well around the nails.

Bones, Joints, and Muscles

We don't think about it while we're young, but as we age we remember the injury from the big football game every time we have pain in that shoulder. Old injuries we incurred in youth often become the places where arthritis lands in our joints.

Here are some simple formulas for soothing those minor problems. Hindsight is good — if we would have known in our 20s that we'd ache in our 50s, we might have treated ourselves better!

Arthritis Poultice for Swollen Joints

Here's the pharmacist's treatment for arthritis. **Note:** *This is not to be taken internally, so label it FOR EXTERNAL USE ONLY and never use it in a tea. All herbs should be dried.*

6 tablespoons mullein leaves (*Verbascum thapsus*)
9 tablespoons slippery elm bark (*Ulmus rubra*)
3 tablespoons lobelia (*Lobelia siphilitica*)
1 tablespoon cayenne pepper

1. Mix all ingredients well, and store in an airtight container in a cool, dark place.
2. To use, take out 2 or 3 tablespoons of the mix and add enough boiling water to make a paste. Spread on a cloth and apply to the affected area. Cover with another warm cloth, such as a small kitchen towel. Use twice daily.

Healing Liniment

Another liniment Jerry Stamps made and sold in his pharmacy was old-fashioned Kloss' Liniment. I've used it on sore joints and muscles, insect bites, and all kinds of little injuries and ailments. I think his formula was inspired by the book Back to Eden, *by Jethro Kloss, but Jerry said his method was a bit different from the original. Here's Jerry's version.*

> 2 ounces powdered myrrh (a tree resin)
> 1 ounce goldenseal powder (or use the dried roots and pulverize them in a blender, measuring after powdering)
> ½ ounce cayenne pepper
> 1 quart vodka

1. Mix all the ingredients in a 1-quart container and shake. Set aside for one week, shaking occasionally. Pour into a smaller bottle and label.

2. To use, pour a small amount into the palm of your hand and then rub into sore area. I've also used this on sores in the mouth by applying three times a day with a cotton swab. *Note:* The goldenseal may stain clothing slightly (although it isn't difficult to wash out).

→ Natural Headache Healing

James Duke, Ph.D., former USDA plant researcher and author of *The Green Pharmacy,* suggests using a combination of bay and feverfew to ward off migraine headache. Studies reported in the *Harvard Medical School Letter* and the *British Medical Journal* both attest to the effectiveness of taking feverfew regularly to prevent migraine attack.

Duke recommends a tea made by pouring boiling water over 4 or 5 feverfew leaves and 1 large bay leaf. Cover with a lid or plastic wrap and let steep for 5 minutes before drinking. Feverfew is also easily taken in capsule form. *Caution:* Pregnant women should not take feverfew as there is a remote possibility of miscarriage.

Living Well

There are no guarantees in life, but we *can* live as if we intend to live forever. If we treat our bodies as well as we treat our cars, eat good food, work at something we enjoy, love and accept being loved, enjoy the process of finding happiness, exercise, and work to improve ourselves each day, we will live the best — and longest — life possible. That's the most anyone can expect, and it seems like a darned good goal for life.

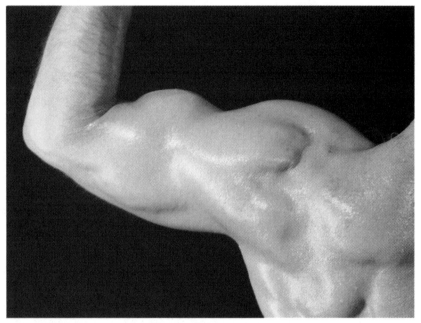

Do what you most love to do in life and you'll be happier, have less stress, and be more fulfilled.

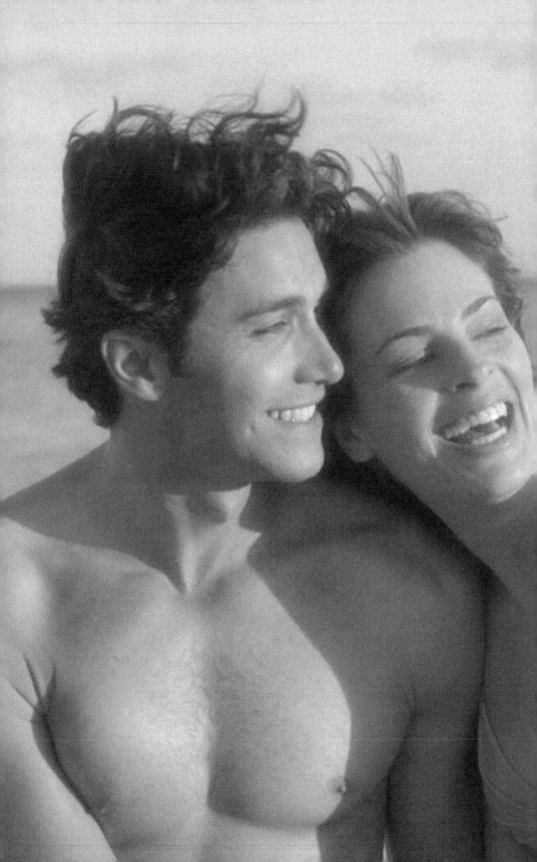

Chapter 2

above the neck

■ DRUMMING IN WILLIAM'S CAVE

It's probably a guy thing, crawling in deep holes in the ground, hanging suspended by ropes, slopping through ankle-deep muck, and crawling on your belly through cracks in the rock so small that the roof gouges your back. But lots of my women friends would disagree, those aspects of caving holding the same appeal for them.

I've been exploring caves since childhood. But it was in William's Cave, more recently, that the "real guy" thing took place. Deep in the hills between the Ozark and Boston Mountain chains, up on the side of a long, steep climb, lies the entrance to William's Cave. It's not officially known by that name, as it's a private place, and suffice it to say that William would like it to stay that way.

The cave mouth has been altered very little since the time of the Louisiana Purchase, walled up just a bit so that there is a doorway locked with steel bars and a padlock. The 16 men who came to the cave ranged in age from the mid-20s to a gray, elderly, and very fit Cherokee gentleman in his late 70s. It was October, a full moon weekend. A few men had brought drums of various kinds, from modest ones that fit nicely in the triangle made by crossed legs on the ground, to tuned drums, to huge wooden drums that had to be laid on their side. The drummer would straddle the drum, sitting firmly on its back to hold it in place with his knees on either side, kind of like riding a horse.

We gathered just as the sun was setting over the line of mountains behind us. This was communing with nature, getting in touch with the caveman inside, each of us anticipating with rising excitement the chance to tap into our primal spirit. It was a personal journey for each of us, a sharing of our bond as men, and great adventure for some.

As darkness descended, William lit a candle and disappeared into the dark cave. Within seconds there was a dull glow inside. We were immediately drawn into the cave, eager for the experience.

The long passage from the mouth wound downward, left and right, around boulders, through low areas where we had to stoop, even across a narrow bridge of rock over a ravine. Small lights, placed behind boulders solely for this event, shone upward but magnified the depth and foreboding of the ravine below. The passage took sharp turns at surprising angles, but always downward, deep into the mountain. Then, quietly, we rounded a bend in the passage and suddenly we were in the mouth of an enormous room.

Roger, one of the first to see it, whispered in an awestruck voice, "My entire two-story house could fit in here with room left over for my yard and driveway!" The floor was mostly flat, rising in the back and leading upward to other passageways and rooms. Tiny crystals of quartz flickered in the veins that ran across the ceiling like lightning across a darkened sky. Most impressive, however, were the enormous onyx columns in the center, 60 feet high and bigger around than two cars parked side by side, appearing to hold up the nearly flat ceiling. The hidden lights among the stalactites and stalagmites that surrounded the columns made the translucent onyx glow as if it were alive, like the sinew of a giant we had just disturbed from sleep.

Further inside on a level area, on several spread-out woven blankets, we men sat, waiting, not knowing what to expect. It's difficult for a group of men to sit, not knowing what is to happen, not being in charge, not in on the plan. Then the drummers began to drum. First it was a slow, uneven rhythm. Each drummer was an individual, not used to drumming in a group, and it was a cacophony of sound, but within a few minutes the larger drums had set the beat and the other drums took up the rhythm.

As the rhythm took on one steady beat, someone turned out the tiny hidden lights, except for a string of small glowing ones deeper in the cave's chambers. Just a faint, distant glow illuminated the cavern. Then those, too, were turned off, and the drums pulsated in absolute darkness.

There is no darkness so severe, so total and heavy, as that felt deep inside the earth. There is no distant star, no glow of a familiar skyline for a point of reference. You can't make out a silhouette, not even of the person beside you, nor see your hands or feet. And I am convinced that in the bowels of the earth you can actually feel the thousands of tons of rock overhead. It's so powerful that it seems the weight of the very darkness itself bears down on you, holding you in place, at once both a secure and a frightening feeling.

As we explored the dark with our minds, straining to make our eyes see what could not be seen, the two enormous drums joined the others. Drums are so primitive, so vital, both quieting and exciting. My heart raced, my mind darted here and there. Would these intense sound waves dislodge boulders and cause the cavern to collapse? Had anyone ever tested concentrated sound waves inside rock? Wasn't it Joshua in the Bible who brought down the walls of Jericho by sound? Wasn't this how Captain Kirk on *Star Trek* freed the captives who were embedded in stone, by using sound waves?

Probably every man was thinking something similar, but all remained silent. Then, as my mind quieted and I gave myself over to the intense and repetitive pulse, my heartbeat seemed to join the drumming rhythm, as well. Later, hours later, all agreed that we felt we had become one with the drums, one with the darkness, one with the earth. We had at once been without body and, at the same instant, a baby in the womb, about to see the world for the first time.

It was a deeply spiritual experience for us, each man finding his strength, his spiritual center in different ways, but not one man of the 16 who went into the cave was left unmoved by the night of drumming. None of us knew how long we were inside, no one wore a watch, and it didn't matter, really. We had been in the cave, one with the drums for several hours, deeply connected to the earth and to our own hearts and minds.

Afterward, each man wandered off to his tent in the ancient oak woods, spellbound, speechless, and lost in the memory of our hearts matching primitive rhythms deep in the womb of the earth.

Caring for Your Body for Life

Women have known for aeons how to care for their skin and hair. Men remain in the dark; we're cavemen when it comes to taking care of ourselves. We bang our heads on cave tunnels, fill our hair and cover our faces with dirt and dust and grime, then expect a fast splash of water to take care of it all. This chapter includes lots of healthy things to do to care for your eyes, ears, hair, and face.

About Face

Men usually don't spend as much time in front of a mirror each day as women do, but that doesn't mean that a man isn't interested in how his face and skin look. It's what other people look at first, our storefront, the hood of our car. We want our skin to remain youthful, to avoid wrinkles for as long as possible, and to stay attractive. The daily activities of work, frowning, stress and worry, sun, pollution, wear and tear of aging, all can take their toll. Here are some ways to keep our skin youthful.

A note about water: For recipes that you are applying to the face as a soak or steam, use bottled water rather than tap water (unless you have a really good deep well or a pristine spring in your backyard). The chlorine in tap water can dry out your skin.

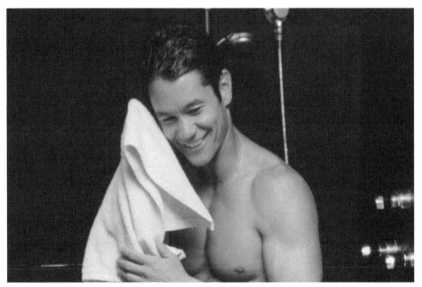

Many guys don't think twice about skin care, but a good skin-care regimen now means the best face possible down the road.

Herbal Face Wash

Most guys run a washcloth over their faces or take a quick shower in the morning to rinse off shaving cream, and call that washing. Here's a way to freshen up old skin. Use this face wash once a week, even once every few weeks, and it will keep your skin cleaner and feeling good. The herbs in this formula are astringents; that is, they help to close the pores and tighten and refresh the skin.

> 2 tablespoons thyme, fresh or dried
> 2 tablespoons mint, fresh or dried
> 2 tablespoons sage leaves, fresh or dried

1. Put the herbs in a small mixing bowl. Pour 2 cups of rapidly boiling water over the herbs, cover with a lid or plastic wrap, and set aside to cool. The hot water extracts the essential oils from the leaves, and the cover keeps the oils from escaping in the steam, falling back instead into the liquid as it begins to cool.

2. Heat about 1 cup of the liquid on high in the microwave. You want it hot, but not boiling (boiling again will evaporate the herb's oils). Soak a washcloth in the heated liquid, then wring it out. Place the cloth on your face for about 5 minutes. Lie back on the bed, the floor, or a comfortable recliner with a warm towel beneath your head, the washcloth over your face. Repeat if it feels good. Refrigerate the remaining liquid for later use. Rinse if you want with cool water, but it isn't necessary.

Sage Steam with Washcloth

This skin treatment couldn't be easier to make. The astringent properties of sage will help tone and refresh your face.

4 tablespoons sage leaves, dried or fresh

1. Bring 2 cups of water to a rapid boil in the microwave or on the stove. While still boiling, pour into a bowl over the sage. Cover with plastic wrap or a lid, and set aside to cool. Strain the liquid, discarding the herbs. Bottle the liquid.
2. Warm 1 cup of the liquid but do not boil. Soak a washcloth in the liquid, then lightly wring it out. Cover your face with the washcloth for 5 minutes.

Screwdriver Face Toner for Oily Skin

A toner is like an aftershave, but with more body and skin-toning characteristics. The vodka is slightly drying, but also removes excess oils. The witch hazel tightens the skin and closes the pores. The orange juice is astringent and healing. Splash on after washing or shaving. Leave it on for a minute or two, then rinse.

Note: *Do not drink this mixture! Witch hazel water is not to be ingested, although witch hazel bark is sometimes recommended for mouthwash and other medicinal uses. Witch hazel in this form (the liquid) is definitely not for internal use.*

4 ounces vodka
3 ounces witch hazel water (the liquid from the pharmacy)
2 ounces fresh-squeezed orange juice

Combine all ingredients and mix well. After washing face normally with soap and water, apply Screwdriver Face Toner all over the face and leave it on for a couple of minutes. Rinse with plain water. This tightens tired skin.

Randy Brandy Face Splash

This face splash is recommended for oily skin. You can double or triple the recipe and bottle it so that you don't have to mix it up each time. For very oily skin, use two to three times per week.

3 ounces brandy
3 ounces vodka
3 ounces witch hazel water
6 whole cloves
⅛ teaspoon ground allspice
About 2 tablespoons fresh orange peel

Combine all ingredients in a jar or suitable container with a lid. Shake and set aside for 1 week to extract the oils and fragrances from the plant material. Don't strain; just pour out a small amount in your hand and splash on like an aftershave lotion. Leave on for about 1 minute. Rinse off with a warm washcloth, and dry as usual.

Keeping the Balance

Skin toners and fresheners are meant to adjust the pH balance of your skin. The skin's pH usually falls between 4.2 and 5.6, and the layer of skin that stays acidic is a protective measure to keep bacteria from growing. If the pH rises to a more alkaline level, bacteria get a foothold and you will experience itching, drying, or other skin irritations. Too much washing with soap, which is usually more alkaline than your skin, can get the pH out of balance. Toners and fresheners are generally more acid than soap, and should be used from time to time after washing.

Gin & Tonic Toner

This is another great splash for oily skin.

4 ounces gin
4 ounces witch hazel water
Peel of 1 whole lemon, cut into
thumbnail-size pieces

1. Combine the ingredients in a bottle or jar with a lid, and set aside for 1 week.
2. Pour out a small amount in the palm of your hand. Spread over your face and leave on for 1 minute. Rinse with a washcloth and warm water. Repeat about every 5 to 7 days to remove oils from the skin. For excessively oily skin, dip a corner of a washcloth in this liquid and use daily.

The Wonder of Witch Hazel

The witch hazel "tree," as it is called in old herbals, is actually a bush and gives us one of the most pleasant, healing astringents available. It's used for all kinds of skin conditions, including bruises, varicose veins, and hemorrhoids. If you have difficulty finding witch hazel liquid, write to the Consumer Affairs Office of the T. N. Dickinson Company (see Resources). The T. N. Dickinson Company has been making 100 percent distilled witch hazel for many years, and can help you find its product. The Vermont Witch Hazel Company is also a good source (see Resources).

Face Lotion for Dry Skin

This lightly scented, simple-to-make lotion makes an excellent moisturizer.

> 4 ounces witch hazel water
> 1½ ounces glycerin
> 1 sprig fresh rosemary (a sprig is a branch,
> about 4 inches long), broken in half

1. Combine all ingredients in a bottle with a cork or lid, and set aside for several days.
2. Shake well, then with your fingers apply a small amount all over your face. Massage in and let dry. Use this every other day to add moisture to your skin.

Chamomile-Cucumber Wash

This combination of herbs and alcohol is excellent for oily skin. To extract the juice from a cucumber, cut one small or half a large peeled cucumber into chunks, removing the seeds. Put in a blender and pulse-blend. With your hands, squeeze out the juice. Save the liquid, and discard the solids.

> ½ cup water
> 2 teaspoons chamomile flowers, dried
> 3–4 tablespoons (approx.) cucumber juice
> 4 tablespoons witch hazel
> 1½ tablespoons vodka

1. In the microwave or on the stove, heat ½ cup of water to boiling. While the water is rapidly boiling, pour it into a small mixing bowl over the chamomile flowers. Cover with a lid or plastic wrap, and let cool. Strain.
2. Mix the cucumber juice, witch hazel, and vodka with the chamomile tea. Refrigerate until ready to use (keeps for 2 to 3 days).
3. To use, pour a small amount of the liquid in your hand and apply with fingers, spreading it all over your skin and rubbing it in. Leave it on for 1 to 2 minutes. With a warm, damp washcloth, wash your face well. Repeat if your skin is especially oily. Dry face as usual.

Face Scrubs

Scrubs are used to clean out really clogged-up skin pores. We're all aging, and as we do our skin gets clogged with dead cells and grime. A good scrub removes the dead cells, gets out the oils and dirt, and tightens the skin, leaving it looking younger and fresher. My advice is that you don't tell your male friends that you're doing this. Just let 'em wonder why you seem more healthy and refreshed.

Face Scrub for Clogged Skin

¼ cup sliced almonds
1 small cucumber, washed, peeled,
   and cut up, most seeds removed
1 teaspoon marjoram leaves, stems
   removed (fresh or dried, but fresh is better)
1 teaspoon cider vinegar

1. In a food processor, blend all the ingredients into a smooth paste. Refrigerate.
2. To use, spread a small amount (about 1 tablespoonful) over your entire face. Massage it in with a circular motion. Leave on for about 5 minutes. Remove with a warm, damp washcloth. Rinse with plain water, and dry as usual.

Almonds for Health

Almonds are used in lots of commercial face scrubs, cleansing soaps, and acne preparations. They act as a gentle abrasive as they impart their mild oil. Almond oil is used in some of the best massage-oil formulas, as it is a gentle and healthy lubricant for the skin. According to a study reported in the *Journal of the American College of Nutrition*, eating almonds can help reduce cholesterol levels. The author of the article, Gene Spiller, Ph.D., suggests eating half a handful of almonds several times a week. So scrub your face with this mixture, then munch on some of these healthful nuts.

Aftershaves

Aftershave lotions are thought of mostly as fragrance, but actually the concoction is primarily meant to close the pores and aid in healing. There are lots of herbs that are useful for the face in a lotion and add pleasant fragrance, too. Plain witch hazel, the liquid form from the grocery or pharmacy, is soothing and healing. Here are some ways for making it even better.

Herbal Aftershave Lotion

The herbs add fragrance and some healing benefits, while the witch hazel is soothing to your skin. All herbs in this recipe should be dried.

> 10 whole lemon verbena leaves
> 1 tablespoon lavender flowers
> 1 tablespoon lemongrass leaf, chopped
>   or cut up with scissors
> 2 teaspoons crushed or chopped spearmint leaves
> 2 teaspoons chamomile flowers
> 4 cups witch hazel water

1. Place the herbs in a 1-quart jar. Pour the witch hazel over the herbs, and put a lid on the jar. Shake and set aside in the kitchen. Shake the jar briefly every day or so for a week.

2. Strain out the liquid and discard the herbs. Pour into a convenient bottle for use in the bathroom. To use, splash the liquid on your face after shaving.

Get into the habit of using a high-quality aftershave to reduce razor burn and help small cuts heal more quickly.

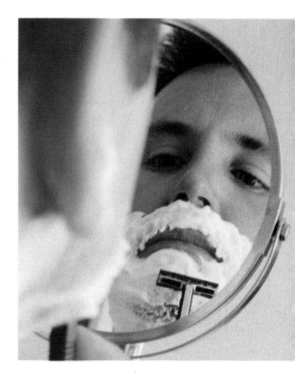

Tropical Breeze Herbal Aftershave

All herbs in this formula should be dried.

4 cups witch hazel water
½ cup roses, rose petals, or buds, or
    any combination
½ cup lavender
Peel of 1 fresh orange, cut in pieces
2 teaspoons whole cloves

Place all the ingredients in a 1-quart jar. Cover with a lid and shake briefly, then set aside. Shake every day or so for about a week (two weeks would be even better). Strain and bottle. Use as you would any other aftershave.

Southern Tropics Aftershave

You'll need to buy the smallest size essential oils for this, but lots of guys like this formula so much that they always keep some on hand.

7 drops bay essential oil
7 drops lemon essential oil
3 drops lavender essential oil
10 drops rosemary essential oil
5 drops lime essential oil
2 teaspoons tincture of benzoin
4 tablespoons witch hazel
2 tablespoons rose water (found in pharmacies
    or via mail order)
1 tablespoon cider vinegar

1. Combine the essential oils with the tincture of benzoin, and shake well to dissolve the oils. Add the witch hazel and shake well, then add the rose water and cider vinegar and shake again. Bottle. Store away from heat and light.

2. To use, sprinkle a few drops in your hands, rub your palms together, and spread the lotion on the shaved area.

Bay Rum Aftershave

Try this fragrant concoction if you enjoy the scent of kitchen spices.

About 15 dry, whole bay leaves

1 tablespoon whole cloves

1 small piece fresh ginger, about the size of your thumbnail (get it in the produce section of the grocery store—the same fresh ginger you use when stir-frying)

1 teaspoon ground allspice (or 5 fresh allspice leaves)

2 tablespoons fresh orange peel

2 cups rum

½ cup water

1. Put all the ingredients in a 1-quart jar. Cover with a lid and shake briefly, then set aside for two weeks. Shake the jar occasionally. Strain out the herbs and bottle the liquid.

2. To use, wet your hands with water, then sprinkle several drops of aftershave onto them (this dilutes the aftershave). Smooth onto your face after shaving.

Mustache Tips

Do you get complaints from your lover about how bristly your mustache is? Try using a dry-hair conditioner on it to soften the bristles. If that doesn't take care of the complaints, let your mustache grow longer. Close-cropped mustaches are more irritating to the person whose face is closest to yours. If you just let the mustache grow a tiny bit longer, it doesn't stick out like a cactus under your nose. Longer hairs are softer hairs and softer hairs mean fewer complaints in the kissing department.

Woodsman's Aftershave

I make this for myself and always vary it a bit, depending on what's available. In this recipe I give the approximate amounts; exact measurements aren't necessary.

Any kind of juniper berries will do. They are the little blue berries found on juniper trees and landscape shrubs, commonly called cedar trees. Fresh berries have more fragrance, but you can use dry berries. I pick some through-out the year and let them dry in a basket on top of the refrigerator. You can also find juniper berries at the health-food store and from mail-order sources. **Note:** *If you gather your own, choose berries from bushes or trees that haven't been sprayed with insecticide.*

⅛ cup juniper berries, fresh if possible
1 sprig (4 inches long) fresh pine needles
    with stem, cut into small pieces
2 tablespoons freshly dried orange peel,
    cut into fingernail-size pieces
5 whole cloves
2 whole allspice berries
1 piece (½ inch long) stick cinnamon
1 piece (1 inch long) sassafras root, the diameter
    of your index finger (optional)
3 ounces witch hazel liquid
5 ounces vodka (or brandy, but vodka has
    less of an alcohol smell)
2 ounces bottled water

1. Place the dry ingredients in a glass or plastic jar. Pour the witch hazel, vodka, and water over the herbs. If the liquid doesn't com-pletely cover the solids, add enough additional vodka and witch hazel to completely cover the dry ingredients. Cover the jar and shake well. Shake jar daily for 10 days.
2. Strain, discarding the solids, and bottle. To use, splash a bit of the liquid on your face after shaving.

→ Quick Fix for Razor Cuts

According to Dr. Robert Kotler, a surgeon in Beverly Hills, any nasal spray that has phenylephrine hydrochloride (such as Neo-Synephrine) will stop the bleeding of razor cuts. You've probably got the nasal spray right in the medicine cabinet, so if you're still putting little wads of toilet paper on your cuts, quit it; there's a better solution! Phenylephrine hydrochloride constricts blood vessels, so the bleeding will stop in 5 minutes — or even sooner.

Cologne

The difference between cologne and aftershave is pretty simple, even though lots of men use both products as an aftershave. An aftershave lotion generally contains antiseptic healing ingredients, alcohol, a moisturizer, and water. Cologne is simply alcohol with fragrant oils, sometimes with a bit of water, not meant for healing but just to make you smell good. This type of fragrance originated in Cologne, Germany, hundreds of years ago and today is essentially an alcoholic solution of citrus oils, generally including neroli oil (an essential oil distilled from orange flowers).

Unfortunately, as we men age, our sense of smell diminishes a bit, especially if we're heavy smokers. And sadly, some men can't tell how much cologne they splash on themselves, so they just slap the fragrance all over. Women seem to know that subtle fragrance adds intrigue, that a little smell goes a long way. But many men believe that if a little is good, a lot is even better, and you can smell them coming halfway down the street.

Here are some cologne formulas that will give a subtle, natural, and pleasant aroma — and you won't smell like a traveling cologne salesman, either.

Historic Florida Water

Florida Water cologne was popular before and during the Civil War. An early form of aromatherapy, Florida Water was used to ease headaches, raise the spirits of a patient in the sickroom, and cover up the fact that people didn't bathe all that often. Bottles of Florida Water were available in drugstores and general merchandise stores on the western frontier, were carried by wagon train down the Santa Fe Trail in the 1840s, and were a mainstay of personal hygiene for cowboys on Saturday night, after the weekly bath.

The recipe for this famous fragrance can still be found in old pharmacy references, such as Remington's Practice of Pharmacy, *1948. The recipe from that book is given here; the measurements are adjusted for making a small amount. This isn't cheap, but good colognes aren't either.*

> 30 drops neroli essential oil (30 drops
>   equals about ⅙ dram)
> 30 drops lavender essential oil
> 1½ teaspoons bergamot essential oil
> 12 drops clove essential oil
> 18 drops cinnamon essential oil
> 30 drops rose fragrance oil
> ⅛ cup orange flower water

1. Put all the ingredients in a glass jar with a lid. Shake to mix, then set aside for one week, shaking daily. Check the scent: If it's too strong, add ¼ cup of bottled water.

2. To use, splash a small amount on the face or body.

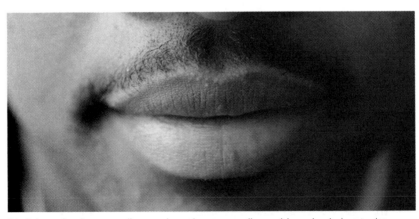

Herb-based colognes will not only make you smell good but also help condition your skin.

Old South Verbena Cologne

2 cups fresh lemon verbena leaves
(or 1 cup dried leaves)
6 whole cloves
2½ cups vodka
½ cup bottled water

1. Crush or mash the lemon verbena leaves, and place them in a glass jar. Add the cloves and the vodka. Put a lid on the jar and shake well, then set aside. Shake daily for one week.
2. Strain and discard the herbs and cloves. Add the water and then bottle. To use, pour a small amount into your hands, rub them together, then apply to the face.

Dry Skin

If dry, flaky skin is your problem, you might want to try calendula oil. You can buy it in the pharmacy as an oil, as a cream, or in an aloe vera base. I like to save the $7 to $10 and make it myself.

Calendula Oil

Calendula has centuries of reputation for being very helpful for troubled skin. It's mildly antiseptic, according to old herbal sources, and soothing. It's pretty amazing on some skin problems and worth trying.

1 cup dried calendula flowers or petals
1½ cups vegetable oil (see box on page 52)

1. Place the calendula in a 1-quart jar. Pour enough vegetable oil over the calendula to cover, top with a lid, and place in a moderately dark place (in the kitchen cabinet or pantry). Shake the jar daily for 10 days. The oil will take on a golden yellow color. You can leave in the flowers, so that the plant's oils continue to go into the vegetable oil, or you can strain out the flowers and discard them.
2. Dip a finger into the oil and massage it into your face. Do this every day; twice a day would be even better. The calendula will begin to heal your skin. You can wipe off the excess after a few minutes.

Using Vegetable Oils on the Skin

Cooking oils are actually acceptable bases for massage oils. You can use a vegetable oil straight from the bottle, or mix it with almond or avocado oil. My preference is a corn–canola oil combination.

Other oils that are pleasant on the skin are peanut and sunflower, both fairly lightweight oils. Grapeseed is one of the most healthy oils to use. But for massage applications, I like apricot kernel oil and sometimes combine grapeseed and either apricot kernel or almond. Those oils are a bit harder to find, but if you plan to use calendula oil regularly, I suggest getting the better grapeseed and almond oils.

Troubled Skin Wash & Tea

This formula is from Jerry Stamps, a pharmacist who lived and worked in Eureka Springs, Arkansas. You'll note that this is both a skin wash and a tea, and is to be used both ways during treatment. It contains witch hazel the herb, rather than the distilled astringent.

1/4 ounce slippery elm powder

1 ounce echinacea root

2 ounces burdock root

1 3/4 ounces wild strawberry leaves

1/4 ounce witch hazel bark (not the liquid astringent)

1/4 ounce chamomile flowers

5 drops orange essential oil

3 drops cinnamon essential oil

1. Thoroughly mix the dry ingredients, then add the drops of oils and mix well again. Take out 1 tablespoon of the material and put it in a glass measuring cup or bowl. Pour 2 cups of boiling water over. Cover with a lid or plastic wrap, and let steep for 5 minutes. Strain.

2. Drink one cup of the liquid in the morning and one in the evening. Also twice a day, pour some, still warm, on a washcloth and apply to your face, leaving it on for at least 1 minute. Don't rinse it off.

Healthy, Handsome Hair

Men are as prone to damaged hair as are women. Oh, sure, women process their hair, using all kinds of toxic chemicals to create curls or to straighten, bleach, dye, or hold it in place, while we men are all-natural, just using water and a bit of shampoo on our hair, right? Yeah, sure. Lots of men use hair colors, gels, or sprays, even if they'd never admit it.

We stick our heads under porches, down drainpipes, inside the engines of big equipment, or in the rafters of old houses, and some of us work outdoors in bright sunlight in all kinds of weather. Many of us live in polluted cities where the air is full of factory and car exhaust smog. Others paint cars or trucks or planes, the fumes penetrating their hair. Still other men work in offices with restricted sources of fresh air. All in all, we treat our hair about the same way we treat our shoes: We wear it, wash it occasionally, but otherwise mostly ignore it, then wonder why it all fell out somewhere along the way.

Here are some healthy things you can do for your hair. The formulas are easy to use and made from simple kitchen and backyard garden ingredients.

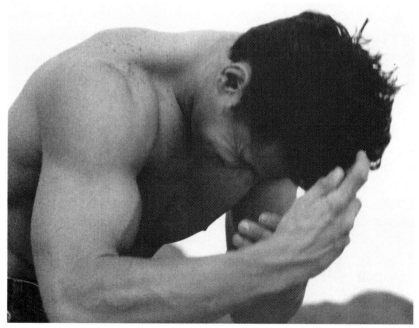

Herbal preparations are great ways to repair damaged hair and keep it healthy.

Herbal Hair Rinses

An herbal rinse gets out the soap residue and leaves the hair feeling and smelling clean. You can make it up in small batches and keep it refrigerated for a few days. I've even made several of these and frozen them for use later. But they're so easy, and so much nicer fresh, that you may just want to do this on a Saturday when you think your hair and scalp deserve a special treat.

Sage with Rosemary Rinse

With regular use, this can darken hair slightly unless you're in the sun a lot. But, sorry, don't expect this to restore gray hair to its former color.

> ¼ cup sage leaves, fresh or dry
> ¼ cup rosemary leaves, or 1 full cup broken up
>   sprigs/twigs/leaves
> 5 cups water

1. Put the herbs in a bowl or pan, and pour 5 cups of boiling water over them. Immediately cover with a lid or plastic wrap, and set the container aside overnight. The next day, strain out the herbs; refrigerate the liquid until ready to use.

2. To use, warm about 1 cup of the liquid in the microwave or on the stove. Don't boil it, just simply warm it. Shampoo hair as you would normally and rinse well. Pour the sage-rosemary rinse through your hair. Leave it in, or rinse it out after a couple of minutes. Your hair will now smell fresh and herbal, and feel clean and soft.

Beer Rinses

Beer rinses have been around for years as a way to make the hair manageable. Beer, after all, is an herbal brew, and maybe it's the herbs that make this work. We do know that all the hops, barley, and malt seem to have some good effects on normal to moderately damaged hair. You might want to try this a couple of times a week, along with taking some hair-repairing vitamins. Just remember to wash out the rinse before you go out; otherwise you'll smell like a brewery! (Or rinse with this before going to your favorite pub, and you'll smell like you belong there.)

Beer Rinse

1 can (12 ounces) beer, fresh or stale

Pour beer through freshly washed hair. Leave in for 20 minutes, then rinse out.

When You Can't Wash Your Hair

Makeup artists who transform movie stars for the screen, as well as nurses in hospitals, know that baby powder, or even plain cornstarch, sprinkled in the hair and then brushed out, removes much of the oil that's in hair. If you're on a camping trip, or even lying flat on your back in bed recovering from something, and find that you're in need of a waterless shampoo, use this easy trick. Dust your hair with a little cornstarch or baby powder, massage it in briefly, then brush it out with a hairbrush. It works in a pinch.

Damaged Hair Repair

If you've sunburned your hair until it looks like a pile of dead sticks, or abused and neglected it in other ways, you should be doing some first aid if you want to keep it on your head. (And if you've done a lot of damage, check with your pharmacy or supplement store and get a suggestion for some vitamins that can help nourish your hair.) Do it now; if you wait until it's falling out, you've waited too long.

Using hair dryers too often is an easy way to damage the hair. Let your hair dry naturally as often as possible. Pat, rather than towel, hair dry. Or here's an alternative that works for some men (except for those anal-retentive guys who never want to be seen unless every hair is perfectly in place). Simply dry the hair with a towel, get dressed as usual, and get in the car without combing your hair. Once you get going (okay, this works better in rural areas than it does in downtown rush-hour traffic), turn the heater and fan on full blast and aim the vents at your head. Open a window if necessary. The warm air blowing through your hair is much gentler than the strong heat of a hair dryer. In about 10 minutes of driving your hair will be dry, and at the first stoplight you can comb it into place. I know it's not for everyone, but it works great for some of us!

Rinse for Damaged Hair

Why egg? Egg is protein, and when combined with beer it makes a healthy rinse that repairs damage and leaves your hair manageable and looking shiny clean.

1 can (12 ounces) beer, fresh or stale
1 raw egg

1. Pour half of the beer in a blender with the egg and pulse briefly. Add the remaining beer and stir.

2. To use, pour this fluffy mess through your freshly washed hair. Wrap your hair in a warm towel and do something else for 15 minutes, then rinse thoroughly with warm, not hot, water. Repeat twice weekly. It really works! (Just remember not to answer the doorbell in this condition, unless you enjoy being laughed at.)

Really Badly Damaged Hair Treatment

Here's an easy way to repair the damage that's already been done.

3 eggs
½ tablespoon mayonnaise

In a bowl, beat the eggs with a fork. Mix in the mayonnaise. Shampoo your hair and rinse. Work the egg/mayonnaise goop completely into your scalp and hair. Leave on for 10 minutes. Rinse thoroughly with warm water, and dry hair lightly with towel.

Specialty Hair Treatments

While there are lots of purported hair-loss remedies made with herbs, I know of none that work reliably. However, there are lots of things a man can do with herbs to keep his hair healthy and in good shape, including healing damaged hair, fighting dandruff, and using maintenance rinses. Here are several of my formulas.

Lemon-Chamomile Rinse

Chamomile and sun exposure are known for lightening hair — not like bleach, but gently. The tips will lighten faster if you use chamomile regularly. If you like the chamomile fragrance and want to use it more often, try just a plain chamomile rinse without the lemon juice and use it daily.

> 4 cups water
> ½ cup chamomile blossoms
> Juice of 2 lemons (don't use bottled lemon juice)

1. In a medium bowl, pour 4 cups of boiling water over the chamomile. Immediately cover the bowl with a lid or plastic wrap and let cool. Strain and add the lemon juice.

2. To use, pour half the liquid through your freshly washed hair (catch it in a pan for another application if you wish). Leave it in for about 5 minutes — leave it in longer for more lightening effects — then rinse. Refrigerate the remaining rinse and use in three or four days. *Note:* Sunlight will speed the lightening effects.

Dandruff Rinse

Dandruff is a problem for some men. In most cases, it's easy to control by getting the scalp pH balanced. If you've got a really bad problem, you may want to use something from the pharmacy, but otherwise I suggest the following.

> 4 cups water
> ½ cup horsetail (*Equisetum hyemale*)
> 2 tablespoons peppermint leaves
> 2 tablespoons cider vinegar

1. In a medium saucepan, bring 4 cups of water to a boil. Add the horsetail and continue boiling for 1 minute. Add the peppermint leaves, then remove the pan from the heat and immediately cover with a lid. Let the liquid set overnight.

2. Strain out and discard the herbs. Add the cider vinegar.

3. To use, warm 1 cup of the rinse to a comfortable temperature. Shampoo your hair normally and rinse well, then pour the Dandruff Rinse through the hair, catching it to reuse if desired. Leave it in and dry lightly with a towel. Use every other day.

Nettle-Mint Dandruff Rinse

The following formula is an adaptation of one from The Herbal Home Spa, *by Greta Breedlove (Storey Books, 1998). She suggests that if the dandruff doesn't clear up in about two weeks, you should see a physician.*

1 cup water
2 tablespoons fresh nettles (see box)
2 tablespoons fresh peppermint leaves
1 cup apple cider vinegar

1. In a small saucepan, bring 1 cup of water to a boil. Add the nettles and peppermint. Remove the pan from the heat, cover immediately, and set aside for 24 hours.

2. Strain, discarding the herbs. Add the vinegar, and bottle until ready to use. Store in the bathroom or in a cupboard.

3. To use, heat 1 cup of plain water and add ¼ cup of the nettle-mint rinse. Pour through freshly washed and rinsed hair. Leave on for 1 minute and rinse out.

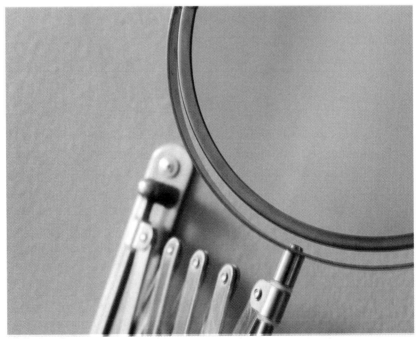

Don't be afraid of checking your hair in the mirror. It isn't vain; it's necessary if you want your hair to be attractive and problem-free.

Beware of Stinging Nettles

The nettle, also called stinging nettle *(Urtica dioica)*, is a very versatile plant. When collecting stinging nettles, first be sure you have correctly identified the plant from a guidebook, such as the *Peterson Field Guide to Medicinal Plants*, by Steven Foster and James Duke. Second, wear gloves! The name stinging nettle gives a clue; it stings like the dickens! I've waded through stinging nettles on camping trips and believe me, the sting lasts for an hour or more and is very uncomfortable. The plant is full of vitamins and other healthy things for your hair, and once heated with the boiling water, the leaves will no longer sting.

Shampoos to Help You Look Your Best

Sure, shampoo is cheap and easy to find, but have you ever read the ingredients on the label? So much stuff! There are ingredients that sound like they belong in the antifreeze mixture of your car's radiator, plus colors to make the shampoo pretty. Besides, it's just plain satisfying to know that you can actually make your own simple shampoo should the need arise.

Fresh Lemon Shampoo for Oily Hair

This is a thinner shampoo, but it still works nicely. It will keep for several weeks if stored away from light and heat.

> 2 cups water
> ¼ cup dried lemongrass (or ½ cup fresh)
> Peel from half a fresh lemon, cut into pieces
> 4 tablespoons liquid castile soap
> 3 or 4 drops vitamin E oil

1. Bring 2 cups of water to a boil. Lower the heat and stir in the lemongrass and lemon peel. Remove from the heat and let cool, covered, for about 2 hours, or overnight.
2. Strain, keeping the liquid and discarding the solids. Add the liquid soap and the vitamin E oil, stir, and bottle. Use as you would any other shampoo.

Shampoo for Oily Hair

Chamomile and gin help remove excess oiliness and leave the hair feeling nice and fresh. Substitute 3 tablespoons of rosemary leaves for the chamomile for a pleasant-smelling shampoo that is better for less oily hair. The shampoo will keep for several weeks.

Castile soap comes in bar form. It's made from coconut oil, and you'll find it in the health-food store or pharmacy's soap section, and in some grocery stores.

1 bar castile soap
4 cups water
3 tablespoons chamomile blossoms
3 ounces gin

1. Grate the bar of castile soap on a vegetable grater or, to be really manly doing this, get out your pocketknife and whittle the bar into little pieces while sitting on the back steps and humming a few bars of the "Battle of New Orleans." You want 2 ounces.

2. Make a chamomile tea by bringing 4 cups of water to a boil. Add the chamomile blossoms and immediately remove the pan from the heat and cover it. Set aside for 30 minutes. Strain, saving the liquid and discarding the chamomile.

3. Heat the liquid again to almost boiling and add the soap shavings, stirring until they are all dissolved. Remove the pan from the heat. Continue to stir, and add the gin. Stir again and pour into a jar or wide-mouth bottle. This shampoo will be similar to the texture of a thick cream.

4. To use, dip your fingers into the container and shampoo with the cream as usual.

Dandruff-Fighting Shampoo

Along with this treatment, you might want to take some hair-repairing vitamins and use a cream rinse once a week.

> 4 cups water
> 1 tablespoon birch bark
> 1 tablespoon peppermint leaves
> 1 tablespoon dried nettles (dried nettles don't sting)
> 1 tablespoon lemongrass
> 1 cup liquid castile soap

1. In a medium saucepan, bring 4 cups of water to a boil. Stir in the herbs, then let cool, covered, overnight.
2. Strain out the herbs and discard. Mix in the liquid soap and pour into a bottle. Use as a daily shampoo. Rinse with Dandruff Rinse (see page 57).

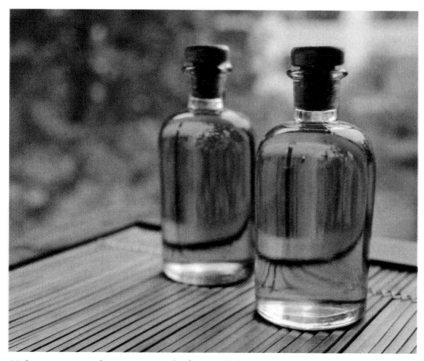

Making your own shampoo is simple, fast, and cheap. Why bother with the chemical-laden stuff when you can have an easy, all-natural version?

Baldness

There are several new treatments for baldness — some that work occasionally, some that never really do much. Herbal folklore is rich with baldness remedies. One of my favorites claims that if you go into the garden at high noon, pick a handful of sage leaves and crush them on your head, rubbing in well, then turn around three times, hair will begin to grow.

Another, from *Young's Great Book of Secrets,* 1878, says, "A most valuable remedy for promoting the growth of the hair is the application once or twice a day of wild indigo and alcohol. Take four ounces of wild indigo and steep it about a week or ten days in a pint of alcohol and a pint of hot water, when it will be ready for use. The head must be thoroughly washed with the liquid, morning and evening, application being made with a sponge or soft brush." I especially like this one because I think it's the basis for the famous, modern-day "hair in a can" you've likely seen on late-night TV. You know the one, where the Ronco guy comes out into the audience and sprays a guy's bald pate with black paint and says, "There, now doesn't that look better?"

The Importance of Eye Care

My father, in his later years, suffered from deteriorating eyesight. He was in his 80s when he began to develop cataracts. We now know that exposure to sunlight without the protection of sunglasses can increase the risk of cataracts considerably. Ultraviolet rays not only hit you directly in the face but also bounce up off the surface of water or snow. To learn more about sunglasses and eye protection, check out the Sunglass Hut (see Resources).

Eat Your Veggies

Diet has a role in keeping your eyes in good shape. Leafy green vegetables, such as spinach and kale, are beneficial. Researchers at the University of Texas in Galveston have proved that kiwi, squash, corn, orange peppers, and red grapes are strong sources of two antioxidants, luetin and zeaxanthin, that possibly prevent, and certainly slow down, vision loss as you age. Frederik van Kuijk, M.D., who was the study's leader, suggests eating at least five servings of fresh fruits and vegetables a day. In addition, bilberry is indicated in maintaining eye health.

Maintaining Good Dental Hygiene

Toothpaste: Now, why would any guy want to make his own? I like to make stuff just to prove I can, just because I'm curious about what's in a product. The Caswell-Massey Company offers an old-timey tooth powder, "like Grandpa used to use." In actuality, my grandpa didn't use tooth powder much; he chewed tobacco. When he was still relatively young, in his 50s, his teeth were so bad that he had them all pulled out and replaced with dentures. Even more than real teeth, I'm told, dentures feel like fur balls unless they are brushed, so he finally got in the habit of using tooth powder. I still have some of the little empty metal cans his powder came in, sitting in my collection of antique bottles.

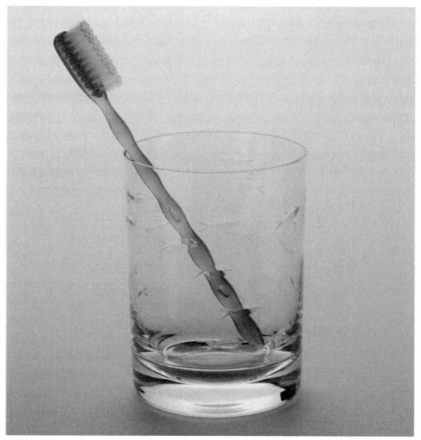

Don't skimp on the brushing and flossing routine; poor dental hygiene is one of the biggest turn-offs for many people.

Mint Tooth Powder

Tooth powder was originally made from baking soda, with salt for an abrasive, along with some flavoring. Here's a simple recipe for making your own.

In place of the spearmint oil, you could also use finely powdered, dried mint leaves. Powder them in the blender along with half of the salt, using about 10 dried mint leaves, either spearmint or peppermint, then mix with baking soda. The mint oil, however, makes a smoother powder for brushing teeth.

> ½ cup baking soda
> ⅓ cup plain, uniodized salt
> 8 drops spearmint essential oil

1. In a small mixing bowl, blend all the ingredients. Store in an airtight container, such as a clean, plastic, leftover yogurt container.

2. To use, pour out about 1 teaspoonful of the mixture into the palm of your hand. Wet the bristles of your toothbrush under the tap, shake off any excess water, and dip it in the tooth powder in your hand. Brush as usual. Your teeth will feel really clean and shiny, and that should make you show off your grin.

Emergency "Toothpaste"

You're on a camping trip and you've forgotten your toothbrush and toothpaste. What to do? Find wild strawberries (cultivated ones work, too). Smash one on your teeth and move it around with your finger. Here's what Sidney Morse said in the 1908 edition of *Household Discoveries, an Encyclopedia of Practical Recipes and Processes:* "The juice of the common strawberry is said to be a natural dentifrice which has the property of dissolving tartar and sweetening the breath." I've used this method several times and found it quite pleasant. Plus, you get to swallow the strawberry "toothpaste" — something that's not recommended with regular toothpaste.

Don't Forget the Ears

Unpiercing your ears? You think that pierced ear hole will grow back in? Wrong, Bucko. The hole fills up with dead skin, but it can still become infected, and it will not close completely. If you want the hole repaired and covered up entirely, a plastic surgeon can take care of it in about 20 minutes for around $350 per hole. If infection occurs, twice daily applications of hydrogen peroxide usually clears it up.

However, holes in the nose, tongue, or lips (or anything else you may have had pierced, such as nipples or penis) aren't as easy to repair. Nose or tongue holes won't grow back. Just think, when you're 85, sitting in your rocking chair in the nursing home, and they bring you a bowl of soup, you can strain out the noodles through the hole in your tongue! To find a plastic surgeon in your area, call the American Society of Plastic and Reconstructive Surgeons (see Resources).

The ears are especially prone to sunburn damage. Dr. Thomas Westbrook Lynch, my dermatologist, recommends using a sunscreen that blocks both UVA and UVB rays. "The sunscreen that is most effective is one that contains Parsol 1789, found in either Ombrelle or PreSun Ultra brands," he says.

If you suffer from earaches, several herbs have been found effective in treating this problem; these include echinacea, garlic, goldenseal, mullein, peppermint, and tea tree oil. Always use caution with ear drops, and do not use them if you have a perforated eardrum.

And what about ear hair? Come on, guys. If you're over 40 and hair's growing out of your ears, no one, regardless of sexual orientation or gender, will find that attractive. If you've got ear hair, get a little rechargeable hair trimmer and cut it out!

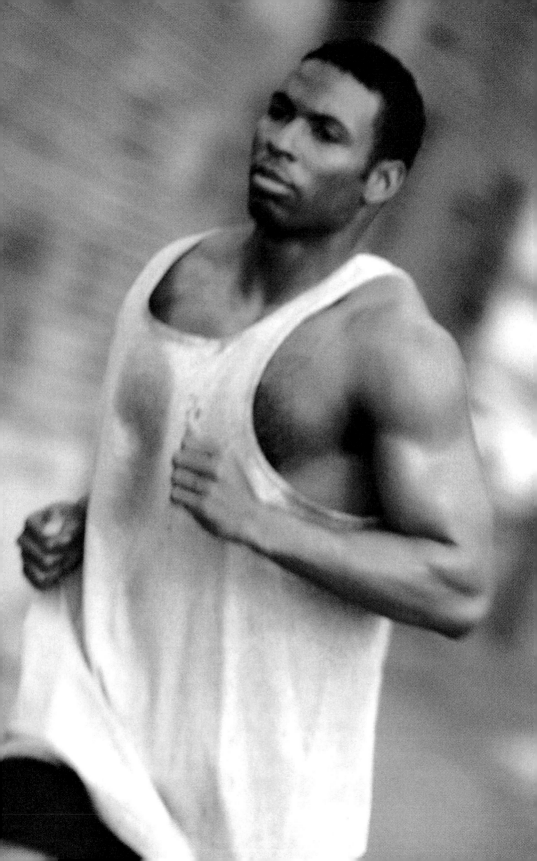

Chapter 3

below the neck, above the waist

▪ GRANDPA AND THE BUFFALO HORN

I keep a buffalo horn in my dining room — it's there for conversation and as a reminder of the past. My grandfather brought the horn back from Oklahoma when he was 17 years old. It's hard to fathom, even now, that my *grandfather* worked as a surveyor's assistant in the Indian Territory before it became the state of Oklahoma.

It's hard to fathom because I'm a baby-boomer, born after World War II, and when I tell people the story of my grandfather, invariably they stop me and ask, "You really mean your great-grandfather, don't you?" We have sizable gaps between the generations in my family, and it really was my grandfather — and I have the buffalo horn as proof.

Grandpa Harper died 13 years before I was born, and maybe because my mother's family always spoke of him with such reverence, I elevated him in my child's mind to the status of a hero, kind of my guardian angel. I used to talk to him regularly, convinced he was hanging around just to listen to my boyhood concerns.

According to my grandmother, Oscar Greene Harper asked his nephew, my grandfather, to accompany him on a trip to the Indian Territory. "Uncle Oscar," as he was always referred to by the family regardless of our relationship to him, was a land surveyor. He was hired by the government to travel to the northern parts of the so-called new territory and mark out the boundaries in preparation for statehood.

Surveying takes at least two people, using strings and measures and tapes and sighting devices. Grandpa was hired to carry things, hold up measuring stakes, pound markers into the ground, look after the horses and equipment, and otherwise be company to his Uncle Oscar. Grandpa Harper, even as a youth, was tall, slender, and muscular, with deep black hair and dark, very serious eyes. He was known in later years as honest almost to a fault and was often called on to settle disputes.

The two set off on horseback, carrying their surveying equipment on a mule. They took along a tent, a coffeepot and a frying pan, a couple of enamel plates and forks, and their bedrolls and canteens. They brought cornmeal, ground from corn they had grown, along with coffee, sugar, several pieces of cured bacon wrapped in paper, a bit of cured ham, lard, and salt. Anything else they needed, they would have to either buy along the way or do without.

In Osceola, Missouri, Oscar and his nephew bought the few remaining supplies they needed, then made their way along the Osage River, following it westward toward the town of Nevada, near the extreme western border of Missouri. From there they traveled on to Fort Scott, a military post on the Missouri-Kansas border, where they met up with other surveyors who were on contract with the government.

For a while the surveyors all rode south together, heading toward the Kansas/Missouri/Indian Territory corner. Soon after crossing into the territory, some split off, heading farther south into what would become southern Oklahoma, while others rode for the central part of the state. Grandpa Harper and Uncle Oscar split from the main group and headed along the southern border of Kansas to their assigned area. They rode west for about three days to the region where they had been assigned to work, found their bearings, and set up a camp.

The land was very different from Harper Community, where both men had lived for all of their lives. The land in Oklahoma was flat and sandy, with scrub oak. Timber for any kind of major construction wasn't available, nor was a river-highway for trade and transportation. Instead, what they found was grazing land where buffalo had been at home for centuries. Native Americans had lived near the buffalo, leading a nomadic life, moving when the herds moved. But those natives were both gone, replaced by woodland tribes from farther east as America moved westward. The Indian Territory had become a holding area, a reservation that had been promised to many tribes that found themselves in the way of westward migration of Europeans.

Those tribes had been moved in a relatively short time in what became known as the Trail of Tears, a forced march under inhumane conditions. The very old and the very young, the weak, the sick, most of them died on that march to the Indian Territory. People succumbed to starvation and, just as often, to complete exhaustion from the forced march in freezing weather spurred on by government men riding horseback. Many Indians were simply shot when they tried to escape their overlords. One leg of the Trail of Tears, I was told as a child, followed along the Osage River and near my father's land where I grew up, and I could see the trail markings that remained.

But the government didn't leave the Native Americans who survived the march for very long on their land in the Indian Territory. Homesteaders were already trying to kill off the "new" Indians and the settlers were petitioning the government to take away even that land. Excursions were made into the Indian Territory to kill off the buffalo, the main food supply for the Indians, without government interference. It was believed that by killing off their food, the Native Americans would either die or travel on. Unbelievable today, it was considered "manly sport" to kill as many of the noble beasts as possible. The buffalo meat wasn't taken, nor were the injured cows or calves even put out of their misery when wounded. It was a gruesome shooting gallery, pushed by greed for land and ignorant hatred of another race.

Grandpa was to tell our family later that it was "a pitiful shame, beyond description," the numbers of buffalo corpses they witnessed when he and his uncle traveled that region. There were still piles of bones and sun-bleached skulls and remains of the huge animals. Grandpa never killed an animal unless it was for food, and he never liked anything to go to waste. He detested the insanity of all the senseless killing and to remember that, he took the horns from a couple of skulls. One, a beautiful black horn with brown stripes, he made into a powder horn to hold gunpowder, and that piece remains in our family today. Grandma always said it should serve as a reminder of the awful way the white people treated the Native Americans.

Uncle Oscar and Grandpa slept out on the open prairie, living off the supplies they brought and the game they killed. If they were injured, they had to repair the scrapes and scratches to their bodies with the herbs they found. Grandpa and Uncle Oscar recognized plants like mullein, dock, arse-smart, burdock, slippery elm, and many more, and knew how to treat their wounds and those of their horses and mule.

Like the time that Grandpa's horse broke its tether during the night and wandered off. Grandpa went looking for the horse. After some walking he spied the horse up on a low rise and took off in a quick run, whistling for the animal. The horse looked up in recognition, just as Grandpa fell over a small mound of rocks. Landing flat on his chest, he had the breath knocked out of him and lay there for several seconds to catch his breath. When he looked up, his horse was standing there, having responded to Grandpa's familiar whistle. Grandpa had a gash in his side from one of the rocks, and Uncle Oscar treated the wound with some of the green salve, made from black dock, goldenseal, and comfrey, they had brought with them.

They relied on their wits and each other for their survival on the plains of northern Oklahoma. Uncle Oscar and Grandpa Harper worked for many months marking off the lines and boundaries, and Harper County, Oklahoma, bears their name to this day.

Learn to Help Yourself

Today, most men don't live on the open plains, out in the elements. We may do so for short times on camping trips, but most of us have other kinds of elements to deal with. We are more likely to have to contend with lack of exercise, injuries from sunburn on a vacation, smog, stress, sitting too long, standing too much, and just the small aches and pains of daily life. Here are some herbal ideas for dealing with the area below the neck and above the waist, and a few tips for good health.

The Chest

Most guys don't pay a lot of attention to their chests unless they're busy bulking up in the gym. But this is an area that houses a couple of major organs — the heart and lungs — and needs extra care.

Treating Coughs and Congestion

What on earth was it that our moms used to rub on our chests when we had a cold? Vicks Vapo-Rub was the weapon of choice for my mother. Any time I had a chest cold or congestion, she'd slather on some Vicks, then she'd cover the salve with a piece of flannel cloth. The story was that the cloth helped the Vicks penetrate the chest, but I always figured it was there either to keep the gunk off the sheets or to keep me from trying to get it off my skin.

Vicks burned like crazy. I remember how hot it was on my tender young skin, just seconds after Mom had spread it on. I'd want to roll and squirm like a puppy in a pile of leaves but Mom would tell me, "Don't scratch it. The Vicks has to soak down deep into your chest so it will help." Eventually the burning would subside, and I would drift off to sleep as the vapors opened my stuffed-up nose.

Chest Rub

The ingredients in Vicks include a combination of eucalyptus and mint oils. Eucalyptus is a fragrant herb, from the leaves of an evergreen tree that grows in warm climates.

You can make your own chest rub if you don't want to use the prepared stuff. The fragrance of the oils will help open your sinuses and the warmth will soothe your chest. The ingredients are simple, and you can find eucalyptus oil in the pharmacy, at the health-food store, or from mail-order sources.

> ½ shot glass cooking oil (canola/corn oil
> combination works well)
> 8 to 10 drops eucalyptus essential oil
> 6 to 8 drops spearmint essential oil

1. Mix together all the ingredients and bottle. Test a bit on your chest or the crook of your arm (the inside, tender part, opposite your elbow). The oil should feel very warm, but not burning, on your skin after about a minute. If it doesn't have that warmth or a distinct fragrance, add a few drops more of each oil; because the strength of essential oils may vary, exact amounts to use will also vary.

2. Dip your fingers in the oil and rub it onto your chest. Cover with a warm cloth and lie down and rest for a few minutes. Better still, get someone to rub it on for you, then ask for a cup of chicken noodle soup!

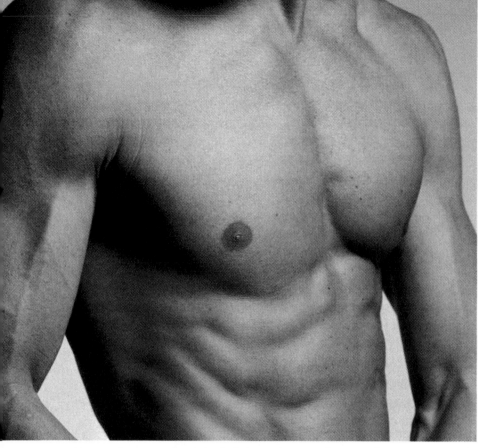

Always take care with any kind of chest ailment, such as coughs or congestion. If they persist, don't hesitate to see a doctor.

Mint-Eucalyptus Steamer

This method of soothing a chest cold doesn't require oil or smearing anything on your skin. Instead, it involves the use of a steam inhalant. If you're miserable with a head or chest cold, you'll probably be willing to try this.

10–12 drops eucalyptus essential oil
8–10 drops spearmint essential oil

Pour 4 cups of boiling water into a pan or bowl. Stir in the oils. Put your head about a foot above the pan, being careful not to touch it, and cover the pan and your head with a warm towel. This will allow the rising steam to surround your head. Inhale the refreshing odor for about 10 minutes. You can do this two or three times a day to help open up the sinuses and help you breathe.

Horehound Cough Drops

My parents ran a small-town grocery store, and they always had horehound cough drops in the pharmacy section. Horehound has been used for countless centuries because it works on coughs. The taste of the drops is both bitter and sweet, but once you get accustomed to the flavor, you won't wait for a cough to pop one in your mouth. Here's a simple recipe for making your own cough remedy out of real horehound herb; it makes about 80 to 100 little cough drops that will keep a year or more. **Note:** *You'll need a cheap (about $3) candy thermometer for this recipe.*

> 8 cups water
> ¼ cup dried horehound leaves
> 4 cups white sugar, plus about 2 cups
>   in a zipper-lock bag
> 1¼ cups dark cane syrup
> 1 tablespoon butter
> 1 teaspoon cream of tartar

1. In a large pot, bring 8 cups of water to a boil, then remove from the heat. Add the horehound and set aside to steep, covered for 20 minutes. Strain, discarding the herb. Butter or spray a cookie sheet (at least 10 by 15 inches, with sides at least ½ inch high), and set aside.

2. To this liquid, add the 4 cups of white sugar, dark cane syrup, butter, and cream of tartar. Cook these ingredients over high heat until they reach the hard-crack stage (300°F on the candy thermometer).

3. Immediately pour the hot candy syrup onto the cookie sheet and spread it evenly with a spatula or the back of a spoon. The candy will begin to cool quickly, so take a kitchen knife and make lines through it in both directions. (These lines will determine the size of the cough drops, so make them small, about ½ inch by ¾ inch.) Dip the knife in hot water from time to time to keep the candy from sticking to it, but work quickly; when the syrup begins to cool, it will go from being a thick liquid to a glasslike, hard candy in just seconds. After scoring, let the candy cool for 5 minutes, or until cool to the touch.

4. Break up the candy along the scored lines. Drop the candy as you break it into the bag of sugar and coat the cough drops on all sides by shaking the bag. Lay the coated drops back on the cookie sheet to dry, uncovered, overnight. Toss them in the sugar again (this is to keep the drops from sticking together) and store them in an airtight container.

Hyssop Cough Syrup

Hyssop is an astringent, and when combined with fennel and honey it helps ease coughing.

¼ cup bottled water
2 tablespoons hyssop (dried flowering top with leaves)
1 teaspoon fennel seeds
1 cup dark, raw honey

1. Bring the bottled water to a boil on the stove or in the microwave. Remove from the heat and stir in the hyssop and fennel seeds. Set aside, covered, for several hours or overnight.
2. Strain the liquid, discarding the solids. Put the honey and herb water in a microwavable bowl and heat slowly on the defrost setting, for about 1 minute, or until the honey is just melted. Stir, let cool, then bottle.
3. For congestion and colds, use 1 teaspoon with each bout of coughing.

Sore Throat Gargle

This formula combines the herbs hyssop and raspberry in a simple gargle. Raspberry (Rubus spp.) leaves are astringent, having a tightening effect on swollen or sore throat membranes.

2 cups water
1 tablespoon dried raspberry leaves
1 teaspoon hyssop leaves or tops
2 teaspoons raw honey

1. In a small saucepan, boil 2 cups of water. Add the raspberry and hyssop, and remove the pan from the stove. Let steep, covered, for 10 minutes. Strain, then add the honey and mix well. Store the liquid in an airtight container in the refrigerator. (It will keep for two or three days; throw out what is not used by then.)
2. To use, warm about ¼ cup of the liquid in the microwave on high. (You want it pleasantly warm but not hot.) Gargle and spit out. You can do this several times a day to ease a sore throat.

Bronchitis and Pleurisy Tea

Pleurisy is an infection of the pleura, the membrane in the chest that covers the lungs and reduces friction during breathing. Pleurisy is painful, often thought of as part of having a cold or flu. My pharmacist friend, Jerry Stamps, gave me the following formula.

Licorice shouldn't be used by those who are on a low- or no-salt diet, as this herb can cause water retention. Substitute 1 teaspoon of fennel seed, which will add a bit of flavor to the mix. The licorice has other benefits beyond flavor, however, and should be used if there are no problems with hypertension or water retention.

> 1 tablespoon licorice root (*Glycyrrhiza glabra*)
> 1 tablespoon plantain (*Plantago lanceolata*)
> 1 tablespoon violet leaves (*Viola spp.*)
> ½ tablespoon yarrow leaves and flowers
> (*Achillea millefolium*)
> 2½ cups water
> ½ teaspoon cayenne pepper or ½ teaspoon
> cinnamon

Blend the licorice, plantain, violets, and yarrow, and store in a plastic zipper-lock bag until ready to use. Add 2 tablespoons of the mix to the water; allow to boil for 3 minutes. Turn off the heat; let steep, covered, for 15 minutes. Add the cayenne or cinnamon and mix well. Drink one cup every 4 hours.

Getting Rid of Heartburn

Tacos, a bowl of chili, lots of beer, some soft drinks, a little plate of chips and dip, throw in a piece of chocolate cheesecake, maybe a giant pretzel with extra mustard, two corn dogs, some beef jerky and a pickled egg, maybe a piece of cherry pie with ice cream and coffee: You're a likely candidate for a good case of heartburn.

Does the menu sound unreasonable? Not really. I've seen men eat worse. You've grabbed a quick bite at the fast-food drive-thru, you head off to the big game with buddies, eat a few snacks there, then stop by your friendly neighborhood bar to toast the team's victory. Afterward, you're invited somewhere to celebrate a birthday. By the end of the day, your belly has had more than its fill. What's a guy to do?

Well, you could begin by not eating all that junk. But if you've already done the deed, try my remedy for heartburn — mint. It won't empty your stomach, it won't undo the calories or the fat and chemicals you've consumed, but it will help with the heartburn. Tums and Rolaids are basically chalk (also touted as "calcium" in the antacid commercials) and mint. Sure, there are other ingredients in some of those stomach-acid equalizers, but generally they are chalk and mint oil, and the active ingredient is the mint.

What if the heartburn persists? You might want to see your doctor if it's a continuing problem. Before doing that, though, you could check in on the Curing Heartburn HotLine (see Resources). That's the automated line at the American College of Gastroenterology, and you'll get answers to lots of your questions about heartburn.

Mint Tea

You can brew up a cup of mint tea and relieve the stomach pain or heartburn without medication. Sound too simple? Check it out and see if it doesn't work for you, too.

If you don't have dried mint leaves, pick a whole fresh sprig (a stem or branch about 4 inches long, with leaves), wad it up in your hand like scrap paper, put it in a cup, and pour boiling water over it. Or use 2 or 3 drops of mint extract from the kitchen spice cabinet in a cup of hot, not boiling, water and drink that slowly.

What about the ribbing you'll take if you're drinking mint tea in front of your buddies? A real man isn't swayed by the kidding of his friends. A real man might teach his buds that he's got a really useful alternative and they can laugh if they want but he'll probably be around to pee on their graves considering what they're *drinking.*

> 1 heaping teaspoon spearmint or
> peppermint leaves

Pour boiling water over the mint leaves in a cup. Cover with a saucer and let the very hot water extract the mint's oils. (This process is called steeping.) Let it steep for about 3 minutes. Drink slowly. You should begin to feel better in a few minutes.

The Stomach

Each of us is responsible for the food that goes into our mouths. Heartburn, upset stomach, weight gain — all are related to what goes into the mouth. Control what goes in and you can go a long way toward a healthier lifestyle. Following are some easy-to-make foods and drinks to help you live and feel better.

Indigestion

Indigestion is defined as difficulty in digesting what has been consumed, and heartburn — the spasming of the lower esophageal or upper stomach muscles — is often a symptom.

Some guys get heartburn out of pure stupidity. They skip breakfast, then get to the office and gulp down several cups of coffee, probably scarfing down a greasy doughnut or two and not eating a real meal until lunch. Then they have heartburn and blame it on the food they ate, instead of what led up to the meal.

As Grandma always said, "Breakfast is the most important meal of the day." That was good in Grandma's time, back when the whole family got up before the sun did, milked the cows, fed the horses, did the

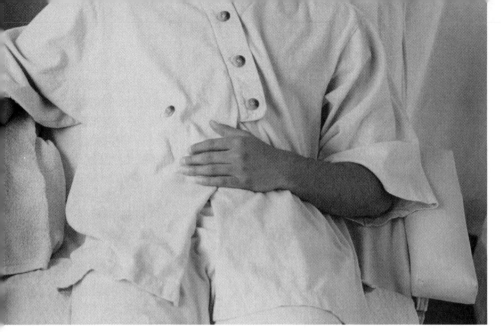

If you don't want to end up with indigestion, watch what you eat. But if the damage is already done, try an herbal remedy for relief.

other chores, then sat down and ate one of Grandma's "meal-for-the-day" table spreads. Back then you could eat two slices of cured ham, three eggs, and half a dozen biscuits with jam along with milk, coffee, and a plateful of fried potatoes, then go out and plow the fields all day and work off the calories. People seldom had upset stomachs or heartburn back then, but they did lots of physical work and didn't gulp their way through fast, gut-wrenching foods, either.

To relieve indigestion, try peppermint or spearmint leaves, fresh or dried, steeped in a cup of hot water (see recipe on page 76). You can even drop two or three leaves (or ½ teaspoon) in your morning coffee. The mint would do you more good without the coffee, but the herb will still help.

To ease stomach gas, Dr. James Duke, retired researcher at the U.S. Department of Agriculture, suggests adding 2 teaspoons of mashed-up fresh dill to a cup of tea (you can use dill seed instead of the leaves). The dill eases the gas and also eliminates bad breath.

The Benefits of Sports Shakes

So what's a health-conscious guy to do about breakfast? We need to eat but we don't have time. We need healthy foods that will give us energy, keep us awake until lunch, make our brains work fast, but not

→

An Old-Fashioned Remedy

An old remedy in *The Indian Physician*, by Dr. Jonas Rishel, which was published in 1828, calls for 3 drops of peppermint oil on a sugar cube as a remedy for hiccups and stomach pain. That's still a good remedy for heartburn. If peppermint oil isn't available, 2 or 3 drops of mint extract from the kitchen spice cabinet works just as well.

require our getting up an hour early to cook. And we need something that's not loaded with grease, calories, or sugar. Here are some of my healthy solutions.

Okay, so sports shakes are really smoothies from the '60s, but if I call them by that name, you won't take them seriously. Juice bars offer smoothies, but who has the time to go looking for a juice bar on the way to work? Besides, they're generally expensive. Here are four recipes that are so easy that you can make any one of them in less than 2 minutes. You can even use your electric shaver or finish dressing while you're making the sports shake. And, even better, the blends of fruit, juice, and yogurt are good for you, they won't make your tummy fat, you'll have energy, and you'll feel 100 percent better than when you were drinking all that coffee and eating those greasy doughnuts. You can even drink one while you drive to work.

The Yogurt Advantage

Think you don't like yogurt? You won't taste it in these shakes, and it's a very good aid to digestion. Choose a plain, low-fat (*not* nonfat — that really does taste awful) yogurt that says on the label, "Made from active yogurt cultures." Use plain yogurt rather than the fruit-flavored ones, which contain more sugar. And always use a clean spoon to dip out the yogurt. Yesterday's spoon, or licking the spoon before putting it in the yogurt, is a great way to grow new, probably undesirable bacteria in the yogurt container.

Sunshine Sports Shake

This shake will make you feel healthy and you won't spend more than a couple of minutes getting breakfast ready. You can even drink it while you drive.

A glob of yogurt (about ¼ cup; exact
   amount is not important)
2 cups orange juice (calcium-enriched if
   you need more calcium)
1 whole banana
1 apple, core removed but peel left on
1 tiny pinch of cinnamon (see Note below)

Place all the ingredients in a blender and pulse-blend for 30 seconds. Pulse a bit more if the apples aren't completely pulverized. Serve with a toasted whole-wheat bagel.

Note: A pinch is a lot less than ⅛ teaspoon. Use a toothpick if you are nervous about measurements; a pinch will fit on the end of a toothpick if you dip the toothpick into the cinnamon *twice*.

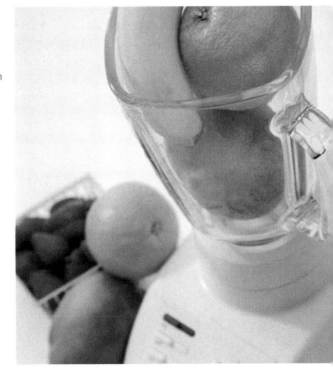

A delicious array of fresh and frozen fruits can be used to make super-healthy, super-tasty sports shakes.

Too-Good-to-Be-Healthy Sports Shake

I like my sports shakes to be as cold as possible. I keep the fruit juices in the refrigerator, and if I'm using fresh fruit at room temperature, I add four or five ice cubes to the mix before blending. Frozen fruit or a frozen banana also helps.

This shake is so delicious, it's hard to believe it's good for you. But one look at the list of ingredients would make even Mom proud.

> ¼ cup frozen blueberries
> 1 whole apple, cored, cut into chunks, peel left on
> 1 banana, fresh or preferably frozen, broken in half
> ¼ cup sliced peaches, canned, fresh, or frozen
>   (about a half peach if fresh)
> Pinch of cinnamon
> ½ cup yogurt
> 1 cup apple juice

Put all the ingredients in a blender and mix well, about 30 seconds. This makes enough for you to have a small glassful while you eat your toast and a little bit left for the commute to work.

How Much Calcium Do I Need?

Women have to be especially careful about getting enough calcium in the diet, but men also need calcium to keep their bones from breaking in old age. To get the recommended amount of calcium, you would have to drink four 8-ounce glasses of milk a day. How about calcium supplements, you ask? According to Bahram Armjandi, Ph.D., R.D., supplements made from the mineral dolomite or from oyster shells are often high in lead, and you don't want to increase your intake of lead.

Is there a better alternative? Six ounces of sardines, bones and all, will give you 650 mg of calcium. One-half cup of tofu provides 450 mg, and canned salmon offers 362 mg per 6-ounce serving. Kellogg's All-Bran cereal provides 210 mg per cup, and turnip greens, kale, and navel oranges all give varying amounts of calcium. The bottom line? Drink some milk and adjust your diet to include calcium-rich foods, then take a supplement if needed.

Papaya-Pineapple Sports Drink

Papaya has enzymes that help you digest food. Even dried papaya is an aid to digestion. But for this recipe, you want to use half of a fresh, ripe papaya; refrigerate the other half for the following day.

½ fresh papaya
½ cup yogurt
1 can (8 ounces) pineapple juice
1 whole apple, cored, cut into chunks, peel left on
Tiny pinch of powdered gingerroot or cinnamon
1 banana, fresh or frozen (preferred)

Put all the ingredients in a food processor and blend for 30 seconds, or until all of the apple chunks are thoroughly pulverized. Serve with a whole-wheat English muffin or toast.

Frozen Fruit

What makes these shakes creamy is the yogurt, and what makes them good is the icy-cold fruit. I keep bags of frozen berries in the freezer in zipper-lock bags. When making sports shakes, I can reach in the freezer and take out a handful of whatever berry I have handy. Raspberries, blueberries, blackberries, and strawberries are all easy to keep around that way. Pieces of melon also freeze well, and bananas freeze especially well. If the bananas I've bought are getting brown, I simply peel the extras and put them in a plastic freezer bag.

Don E.'s Oatmeal Power Drink

My friend Don E. has the most well-defined, nearly perfect body of anyone I have ever known. He's not a fanatic, but he does watch what kind of food goes into his mouth. I asked him what he eats for breakfast and he said he can barely stand food early in the morning. "But I work hard and have to have something to give me energy," he said. Sports shakes, made of juice and fruits, are his main breakfasts. "But," he said, "sometimes I need something heavier that will stay with me until noon. So about three days a week, on average, I make what I call my oatmeal power drink."

I've adjusted his recipe slightly to flavor it, and with the touted cholesterol-fighting effects of oatmeal, this is even more attractive for guys who want a fast but healthy breakfast. This makes a tall glassful and is cold and ice creamy.

> 1 cup raw oatmeal (I use quick oats, but Don E. uses whole, rolled oats or a combination of the two)
> 1½ cups 2% milk
> 4 or 5 ice cubes
> ⅛ teaspoon vanilla
> ½ banana, fresh or frozen

Put all the ingredients in a food processor and pulse-blend three or four times to break up the ice. Blend for about 30 seconds more.

Get a Blender!

If you're serious about healthier eating and don't have a good blender, consider upgrading. Get something with real power, something strong enough to turn apple chunks into pulp in about 10 seconds. I use a commercial-type Osterizer (like they have in most bars). It has a stainless-steel blender bowl and comes apart for easy cleaning. I can grind coffee beans in seconds, or crack soybeans for vegetarian chili. More important, if I fill the blender bowl with fruit, some of it frozen, it doesn't grind and groan, but instead turns everything into liquid in a flash. It takes only seconds to make a sports shake, and only a few more seconds to wash the blender.

Cuts and Bruises

Back when I was in the Air Force and stationed in Texas, I would drive 8 hours home to my parents' house occasionally on weekends. Some of my friends and I would get together and go caving. One particular time we wanted to get an early start, so we drove to an abandoned farmstead and camped out for the night in an old barn.

After a quick breakfast, we headed through a field and along a shallow creek. We carried ropes and flashlights and crossed the creek on a fallen log. The cave was halfway up a bluff face and we eagerly began to climb. All of the guys were climbing ahead of me; one was already up to the plateau where the cave was thought to be, the other two were just above me. Suddenly one guy's foot slipped, dislodging a rock about the size of a large cantaloupe. It bounced and tumbled, then slammed right against my side, nearly knocking the breath out of me. Luckily, I had a good grip on a sapling that was growing out of the bluff and clung to it until I could regain my breath and my footing.

We continued our climb, with me being more wary than ever of loose rocks overhead, and explored the cave. The next day I was awfully sore, with no broken bones, no torn skin, but a really, really sore bruise. It was on that trip that I learned about the healing herb arnica.

The Healing Power of Arnica

Arnica *(Arnica montana)* is a very useful herb for treating bruises. Native Americans used a variety of the plant and even Commission E, a body of experts that advises the German government about herbs, attests to the herb's effectiveness for that purpose. It was also a favored herb by my pharmacist friend Jerry, and he used it in several of his sore muscle and bruise medications. *Caution:* Arnica is not to be taken internally, or used on cuts or bruises that have broken skin.

There are several ways to use arnica. One method that is recommended by James Duke, Ph.D., is to use 1 teaspoon of the dried plant to 1 cup of boiling water. Pour the boiling water over the herb, cover with a lid or plastic wrap, and let steep until completely cool. Then you simply soak a cloth in the liquid and lay it on the wound. Arnica is also useful in treating sprains, dislocations, and joint problems.

Bruise & Sore Muscle Oil

James Green, in The Male Herbal: Health Care for Men & Boys, *suggests making an arnica oil to keep in your tackle box or toolbox for just such injuries. He recommends using equal parts of St. John's wort, arnica flowers, and calendula flowers in an oil infusion. I've adapted his suggestions into my own easy formula.*

¼ cup sunflower–canola oil blend
1 teaspoon arnica flowers
1 teaspoon St. John's wort
1 teaspoon calendula flowers

1. Warm the oil in the microwave on high; you want it hot, but not boiling. Combine the herbs and hot oil in a small jar or container. Put the lid on securely and shake briefly.

2. Set aside for 10 days, shaking the container daily. Strain out the herbs and discard, saving the oil. Bottle and keep handy, but store away from heat and light.

3. To use, rub a small amount of the oil on the bruised area twice daily, massaging it in gently.

Bruise Salve

You can also use the above oil to make a salve, which is less messy.

2 tablespoons beeswax shavings
4 tablespoons of the Bruise & Sore Muscle Oil
(see recipe above)

1. In a small, microwavable container, heat the beeswax to almost melting on medium setting.

2. Warm the herb-infused oil in the microwave and add it to the melted beeswax. Microwave again on low for about 25 seconds, or until the wax is completely melted. Don't allow the oil to bubble or get too hot, as the herbs will vaporize out of the oil.

3. Stir the mixture and pour it into a small container to set up. As soon as it cools, the salve is ready for use. Spread some on bruised places or sore joints several times a day. The salve will keep for a year or more, and doesn't need to be refrigerated.

Arnica Salve

Keep this salve in a handy place to apply to bruises. The same holds for this as with other arnica preparations — use only on bruises, not on an open wound or cut.

> ¼ cup petroleum jelly (such as Vasoline, or you can use commercial Aquaphor Salve Base from a pharmacy)
> 1 tablespoon dry arnica, finely chopped
> 2 tablespoons beeswax

1. Place the petroleum jelly in a small microwavable container and heat on the lowest setting. Heat in short sessions, 10 to 20 seconds at a time, until the petroleum jelly is completely melted.

2. Add the arnica and mix well, then set aside overnight.

3. Heat the petroleum jelly again the same way. When melted, strain out the majority of the herb with a tea strainer (this is optional).

4. Cut up or shave the beeswax into small pieces and add to the petroleum jelly. Melt all in the microwave on the lowest setting. When melted, dip a spoon into the liquid and let it set up in the air, about 1 minute. If the salve seems too runny, heat the liquid again briefly and add a few more beeswax shavings. Stir briefly, then pour into a small container and cover tightly.

5. To use, gently massage the salve into painful bruises.

Chickweed First-Aid Salve

An excellent herb that you can use on cuts, on scrapes, and for other first-aid needs where the skin is broken is chickweed. Yes, plain old chickweed (Stellaria media), the low-growing weed that you probably spray your lawn for in the spring, is a very good first-aid plant. Simply gather chickweed in late winter or early spring and dry it. Chickweed salve is great to keep in the tackle box.

> 3 tablespoons sunflower–corn oil blend
> 2 tablespoons finely chopped dried chickweed
> 2 tablespoons beeswax shavings

1. Heat the oil in the microwave on medium so it's hot but not boiling. Remove from the heat and stir in the chickweed, then set aside overnight.

2. Strain out the chickweed and save the oil. To the herb-infused oil, add the beeswax shavings and warm again in the microwave, being careful to heat it just enough to melt the beeswax. Mix well and pour into a small container.

3. Apply the chickweed salve to scratches, scrapes, small cuts, and small wounds of almost any kind.

Soothing Lavender Oil

Lavender oil is an excellent insect-bite remedy. Some essential oils shouldn't be applied "neat," meaning directly from the bottle. Lavender oil, however, can be applied that way and helps relieve the itch of insect bites. Even mild rashes are helped by this oil.

According to the latest research on mosquitoes, as reported on National Public Radio, insects are twice as likely to be attracted to people wearing the color blue as any other color. If this is true, you could reduce your chances of being bitten by 50 percent by wearing anything but blue clothing. So try it, but keep a little vial of lavender oil handy for the next time you get a bite or an itch.

The Back

Most guys know and ignore the advice to be careful with their backs. But the back is one of the most important parts of the body, as it provides the necessary support for almost all physical activity. The back is also one of the easiest areas to injure, what with all of our bending, stooping, hunching, and lifting. It's not surprising that back pain is a major complaint among men.

Dealing with Back Pain

There are many kinds of back pain, and just as many reasons for it. I'm no expert on most, but I have become a kind of self-styled authority on one particular problem. When I was about 15 years old, I worked outside of town for farmers in the summer, instead of working in my parents' grocery store.

One summer a farmer hired several of us young guys to help him put up hay. I evidently was the strongest-looking because he assigned me the job of putting the hay in the barn. The problem came when the farmer was rushed and had trouble with his equipment. The hay bales got heavier and heavier, some of them topping 90 and 100 pounds, I later learned (when the farmer came to apologize for my injury). I had to lift the bales, then throw them up and over my head, high onto the stacks of hay. Each wagon held 50 to 75 bales. I was young and naïve. I wanted to please my employer and earn my wages and thought that if I complained, I'd be fired. I probably only weighed 125 pounds myself, so I was lifting and throwing bales that weighed almost as much as I did, and I just wasn't used to that kind of work.

I tore ligaments in my back, and that caused my muscles to spasm, or so the doctor said. I had to quit that job and suffered for three years after that, going to numerous physicians without finding relief from the intense pain. I couldn't sleep, had to make adjustments to my bed, and had difficulty sitting in class on days when the pain was intense. Finally I went to a chiropractor, who used heat treatments and massage. Then I began to heal.

I didn't have any more serious problems in college or in the military. But when I was in my 30s, I injured myself again. As a landscape architect, I often got physically involved in design projects. On one particular job, a public garden, stone masons were not available to carry out the rock work I had designed as part of the gardens, and I chose to do the work myself rather than delay the job's completion.

This particular project entailed many low, curving walls and some fieldstone sidewalks — which meant working on my hands and knees. After the fourth or fifth day on my knees, I was in serious pain. I had to see a doctor, who gave me pain medication. I've never dealt well with pain medicines — they always put me in a stupor, and that was the case then. I couldn't work and take the medicine, so I thought I could just tough it out.

Unfortunately, I had torn the ligaments from my old injuries, and in the space of a week was unable to walk without support. I spent the next two months in bed and again tried all kinds of medical advice. I went to several back specialists and a sports injury clinic, but none could offer any real help beyond something for the pain. I spent a miserable summer and fall, unable to sit at my drawing table, unable even to stay out of bed for longer than a few minutes.

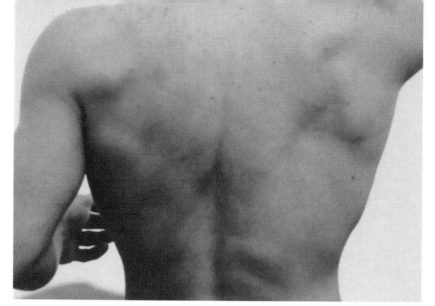

The back is one of the most important — and most neglected — parts of the body. Treat yours right for a lifetime of pain-free activity.

A nurse friend told me to see her general-practice doctor, so I went to see him. He asked questions about how I got my injury, where it hurt, and how it reacted. He asked what I had tried and what kinds of specialists I had been to. Then he told me he thought I wasn't breathing when I worked.

I remember my reaction — I was insulted. "Surely," I thought to myself, "I know enough to breathe." But he kept talking. He explained that when people are in a certain position, like on their knees, they hold their breath when they concentrate. "Lack of oxygen in the blood means that the muscles are more likely to spasm, and the pain will return," he said. "It's like yanking on an already tight rope. Something has to give, and what gives will be the old injured places. Once that starts, you're back dealing with the pain."

The next thing he said to try was to lie flat on my back twice a day for 20 minutes. He pulled a model of the spine out of his desk drawer and showed me how the position would relax the vertebrae where my pain was located. "Try both of these things — intentional breathing and lying on your back, no pillow, just flat on the floor twice daily for 20 minutes. I think you'll be surprised at the results," he concluded.

A pharmacist friend had recommended that I take valerian (an herb known to relax muscles) during the day and again at bedtime. I took his advice as well and started using the valerian capsules. I continued seeing my chiropractor for electrotherapy treatments to relax the injured muscles, and I took the doctor's advice and started breathing and lying on the floor. I was amazed at the changes in my back. The pain began to diminish, the tears at the ends of the ligaments started to heal, and I could both sleep better and resume my work. I began doing specific exercises to improve my back muscles and have had little trouble in that area for many years.

Back Soak

Here's a helpful soaking bath for back pain. I used it many times during my own struggles, and still soak in a tub of hot water with this mix after a long day in the garden.

> 1 cup whole rosemary
> 1 cup whole thyme
> 1 cup whole marjoram
> 1 cup shavegrass, cut into pieces
> 1 cup calendula flowers
> ½ cup arnica flowers (omit if you have a cut or an open wound)
> 2 cups Epsom salts

1. Combine all the ingredients and store in an airtight container.
2. To use, pour a full cup or cup and a half of the mix into a drawstring bag. Or put the mixture in the middle of a washcloth, pull up the corners and sides, and tie firmly with a strong rubber band. Pour 4 cups of boiling water over the herb bag, and let it steep for 10 to 15 minutes. Pour the bag and the bath tea into a tub half-filled with comfortably hot water. Soak for 10 minutes. Squeeze out the water from the herb bag and let dry for a second use.

Relieving Aches and Pains

During the time that my back was giving me problems and I was learning to deal with the torn ligaments and muscle spasms, I was introduced to a chiropractor in a nearby town. I thought his prices were too high and often balked at going to see him on a regular basis.

Stress and worry can make muscles tense, and tenseness can revive old injuries. When I was running a landscape nursery, I had about a dozen employees, mostly college-age students and a couple of sky divers. Several times during those years, when things got tense and just didn't go well at work, my employees would get together to discuss the situation. Sarah, one of the sky divers, was usually designated to inform me of their decision. The conversation would go about like this: "Jim, ah, I don't know exactly how to say this, but, ah, well, we all took a vote and we think it's time you go back to see Dr. Ron."

Usually I would resist: "Too much to do," or "I have to be here to see to this or that." And always I'd end with, "Anyway, it's too late to get an appointment now."

"Oh, I've already taken care of that. Dr. Ron can see you at 1 P.M. We can handle things here, and we've canceled your other customer appointments."

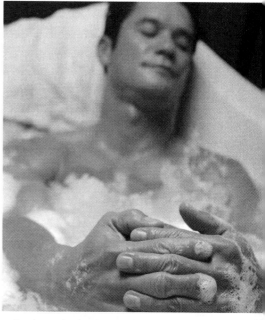

A hot-water herbal bath will do wonders for a strained, tired back.

My resistance broken, I'd give in and make the trip to see Dr. Ron, grumbling all the way. After I was there, I'd wonder why I had been so reluctant.

Dr. Ron's technique was just about perfect. There was a little alcove sitting room where I would wait for my appointment. Another client might be ushered out, then I was invited into the peaceful treatment room.

Soft music was playing. Next I was invited to lie down on a softly padded massage table. Any discussion of soreness or problems was taken care of at that point. Then, for the next 30 minutes, Dr. Ron massaged my muscles with warm oil. It was almost like going into a trance, or experiencing deep meditation. There was only the quiet music, the very warm, comfortable room, and the firm and soothing massage without any conversation or interruption.

Then, after my muscles were completely relaxed — as relaxed as warm honey dripping off a spoon in summer — Dr. Ron would perform his chiropractic adjustments. A soft, fluffy sheet would be pulled up over my naked body and I would be left alone for 15 minutes to rest, relax, or sleep. Coming out of a treatment, I would feel like my feet didn't quite reach the floor, as if I were still floating somewhere on a warm cloud. It was amazing how just that brief time of relaxation and massage could change my mood, lift my spirits, and revitalize me.

Making Your Own Massage Formulas

Dr. Ron relied on my pharmacist friend Jerry for mixing many of his massage oils. Some clients even had specialty blends made up just for themselves when they saw Dr. Ron. An all-natural massage oil is one of the best sore-muscle treatments around when properly used. Here are the formulas for some of those soothing massage blends; the oils are light, suitable for most skin types.

Jerry's Massage Oil

This is one of Jerry's personal massage oils that he took along when he visited Dr. Ron. His soothing, fragranced massage oils were ahead of their time, before aromatherapy became popular. I've had massages many times with this oil and it leaves me relaxed and refreshed, both from the massage and from the relaxing aroma.

2 ounces almond oil
2 ounces sesame oil
10 drops lavender essential oil
10 drops rosemary essential oil
20 drops lime essential oil
20 drops orange essential oil

1. Mix together all the ingredients. Pour into a plastic bottle with a dropper or squirt applicator top, and shake.
2. Squirt several drops on the area to be massaged and rub in well.

Warming It Up

Massage therapists keep their massage oil in a container of very warm water to keep it at a temperature pleasant to the naked skin. Warm the oil, warm the room, warm the massage therapist's hands, and it will relax the person getting the massage.

Satan's Oil

Another of Jerry's formulas, this one is warming and invigorating. The ingredients may seem a bit odd, but they warm the skin. If it's too warm for you, cut the blend with more olive oil. This is very pleasant for a warming massage in winter. It's also useful for backache, tired muscles, sore feet, and even a strained back. Satan's Oil can also be an erotic and fun massage oil; just be cautious when putting it on sensitive areas. Try a tiny spot first, and don't get it in your eyes.

    8 ounces olive oil or sunflower oil, or a
       mixture of the two
    1 teaspoon cayenne pepper
    2 ounces synthetic wintergreen essential oil
    1 ounce camphor
    1 teaspoon kerosene (use the best grade of
       unscented lamp oil)
    1 teaspoon turpentine
    1 teaspoon cider vinegar

Mix together all ingredients and bottle. Shake the contents well, then pour a few drops on body parts chilled from being outdoors or other areas to be massaged. Massage in.

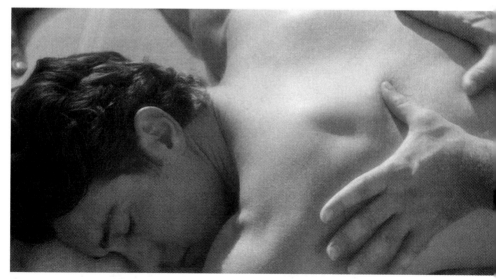

If you can afford a professional massage from time to time, definitely get one. If not, ask a friend or partner to help you out when your muscles are aching.

John's Extra-Special Massage Oil

Jerry's files are full of tantalizing formulas but, of course, there's no information about the people they were made for. We have no idea who "John" is, but this is an excellent, fragrantly erotic blend that is soothing, exciting, and pleasant on the skin. Try it out with someone special, giving each other romantic massages.

> 4 ounces almond oil
> 10 drops orange essential oil
> 10 drops lime essential oil
> 5 drops cucumber essential oil
> 5 drops vanilla essential oil
> 2 drops cinnamon essential oil

Mix together all ingredients. Pour into a plastic bottle with a squirt applicator. Squirt a few drops onto the skin and massage in well.

David's Massage Oil

David was a very talented masseur in the neighborhood who gave excellent, deep-muscle massages. This is David's special blend. It's a bit expensive due to the number of ingredients, but it's so good that you'll want to make it for very special occasions.

Note: *If you have difficulty finding any of the plant oils (other than almond and apricot kernel, which are essential to the formula), you can leave it out, as the other ingredients are mostly for scent.*

> 2 ounces almond oil
> 2 ounces apricot kernel oil
> 5 drops sandalwood essential oil
> 5 drops snowpea essential oil (or substitute
>   5 drops lemon balm essential oil)
> 5 drops balsam essential oil
> 10 drops rose oil (or use rose fragrance oil
>   as a substitute)
> 3 drops vetiver essential oil
> 3 drops rosemary essential oil
> 2 drops lime essential oil
> 5 drops sequoia essential oil (or substitute
>   3 drops cedar essential oil)

Mix together all ingredients and bottle. Shake first, then sprinkle several drops on the areas to be massaged.

The Importance of Skin Care

I remember as a teen how much I wanted to tan. In summers I worked during the day for farmers out in the country, going without a shirt and hat. I didn't want to be pink; I wanted to tan, so on weekends I'd lie in the sun for even longer periods.

When I was 16, my best friend, Gary, and I went on a two-day float trip down the river. We took along our bedrolls, fishing gear, a little food, the boat, and what we were wearing. We both wore swim trunks and shoes, no shirts.

We paddled downriver all the first day, fishing as we went, swimming now and then, but all the time out in the full sun. I began to feel like I was getting sunburned during that first day but Gary was just getting darker. Although the sunshine off the water was burning my skin on all sides, I thought that, surely, this time I would tan. Night was a relief, cooling and soothing.

The following day I spent all of daylight on the water and my sunburn was looking really bad. My thighs, too, were deeply red and burned. By the time we had paddled upriver and returned home, I was sick and having chills. I went to bed. My mother rubbed some kind of soothing cream over my back, chest, and arms. By the next day I was feeling really awful, still with chills and now with an upset stomach. I spent that day in bed. In a few days I began to look like an old board with a bad paint job as the skin peeled off. "This time I'll be tan underneath," I remember thinking. Of course, I wasn't.

I managed never to burn myself like that again, but over the years I've damaged my skin several times. Now I'm paying the price with annual trips to the dermatologist to remove sunspots that are the results of that early damage. The float trips and long hours working out in the summer sun seemed so healthful back then. Sunshine was good for the body, we believed. Now we know better.

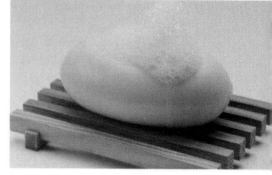

Body odor is a reality some guys don't like to own up to. Do yourself (and your friends) a favor by practicing good hygiene in combination with a healthy, varied diet.

Dryness and Acidity

Healthy skin is on the acid side, pH around 4.2 to 5.6, and this acidity stays on the mantle of the skin. It's a natural protection, something we humans have evolved to keep bacteria from growing on the skin. But most bath soaps are on the alkaline side, and that can cause problems. Dr. Thomas J. Stees, D.O., F.A.C.O.I, the chairman emeritus at the Department of Internal Medicine at the Oklahoma State University College of Osteopathic Medicine, told me, "Men bathe too often, with the wrong kinds of soap." When I asked him to explain, he told me that he has seen many patients over the years who are suffering from what's commonly called "winter itch" — dry, flaky, itchy skin that is more prevalent in the winter.

Tips for Moisturizing Your Skin

"So what should a guy do to prevent winter itch?" I asked. Dr. Stees suggested showering only once a day, less if sweat and body odor isn't a problem. Between times, just wash below the belt, under the arms, and the feet, then use a moisturizing lotion. He also says, "Using Dove soap, which has moisturizers, can also help. It's what I use to keep my skin from getting too dry. It also helps to use a humidifier in the house in winter to keep more moisture in the air."

Greta Breedlove, in her book *The Herbal Home Spa,* says, "If you have itchy skin, be especially careful to avoid using soap excessively, bathing in a tubful of soapsuds, and overmoisturizing your skin. All of these practices interfere with your skin's ability to maintain its natural pH."

→ **Fast Facts**

Years ago I heard someone say, "A good birthday suit is never out of style." The skin is the largest organ of the body, the most sensuous, the most tactile and responsive. An average-size man has about 19 square feet of skin, weighing somewhere around 7 pounds and varying in thickness from $1/32$ to $1/8$ of an inch. Skin is 98 percent protein, and 1 square inch contains approximately 9 feet of blood vessels, 250 to 300 sweat glands, 12 yards of nerves, about 600 nerve endings, 30 small or large hairs, and 40 or so oil glands.

Green Elder Balm

My friend Gayl Bausman, who's been making soaps and lotions for 20 years, shared this formula for a healing, easy-to-prepare moisturizing lotion.

"This is a wonderful moisturizer," says Gayl, "and is effective for burns, bites, bee stings, and even smoothing on poison ivy."

> 4 ounces fresh elderberry leaves (Sambucus canadensis), or 2 ounces dried, chopped
> 1 pint almond or sunflower oil
> 1 ounce beeswax

1. Heat the leaves and oil in a double boiler, covered, over medium heat for 1 hour. Do not boil.
2. Strain out and discard the leaves. Shave the beeswax with a knife to speed up melting and combine that with the warm oil. Continue warming the oil until the wax is melted, stirring well to mix. Pour into a bottle or other suitable container.
3. Dip your finger in the lotion, or pour out a little in your hand, and massage it into the affected places on your skin.

Winter Moisturizer for Dry Skin

Here's another excellent skin moisturizer. It's good for the ankles, knees, feet — any area of skin that is dry. Shake before each use, and keep it refrigerated.

> 2 ounces avocado oil
> 2 ounces almond oil
> 1 ounce plain (not toasted) sesame oil
> 1 ounce wheat germ oil
> 2 teaspoons liquid lecithin
> ½ teaspoon vitamin E oil
> 6 to 8 drops spearmint oil (optional)
> 8 to 10 drops rose fragrance oil (optional)

1. Combine all ingredients except the spearmint and rose oils in a microwavable container, and heat on medium until lightly warmed (but not boiling). Stir in the spearmint and rose oils and pour into a bottle that has an easy-to-use applicator top.
2. Shake well, then pour a few drops onto your palms. Rub together and smooth on affected areas. Apply daily for smoother, less itchy skin.

Protect against Sun Damage

I asked my dermatologist, Thomas Westbrook Lynch, M.D., P.C., and Diplomate of the American Board of Dermatology, what he considered the three most important things a man could do for his skin. His immediate answer was, "Sunscreens, sunscreens, and sunscreens! The vast majority of cutaneous problems we see in men are related to sun-induced tumors, both premalignant and malignant. Basal cell carcinoma is the most common cancer that Caucasians in this country have. On an annual basis, they are more common than the total of all other cancers."

He went on to say that those cancers are due predominantly to sun exposure, which is the cumulative radiation damage that starts in infancy. "Risk factors include being fair-skinned, blue-eyed, of Scotch, Irish, or English descent, and out in the sun a lot. Simply put, the fairer the skin, the greater the risk," he said.

You can cut down on your exposure by wearing tightly woven clothes if you know you're going to be out in the sun for a while. To give you an idea of the difference in sun protection found in various articles of clothing, *Men's Health* magazine says that a standard white cotton T-shirt has a sun protection factor (SPF) of 7, while regular blue denim, like Levi's, has an SPF of 1,700.

Which Sunblock Do I Buy?

The second question I asked Dr. Lynch was his suggestions for choosing a good sunblock. "Use a sunscreen that blocks both UVA and UVB rays," he said, "both of which are damaging. The chemical sunscreen that is the most effective is one that contains Parsol 1789, and two sunscreens that contain this chemical are Ombrelle and PreSun Ultra." He told me again, although I've heard it annually for a quarter of a century, "The most important thing in using sunscreen is to apply it first thing in the morning so it binds to the skin, and do it daily. Remember that on a cloudy day in the winter, the incident radiation hitting the skin is only reduced by 50 percent, so use it summer and winter."

Dr. Lynch continued, "The higher the sunscreen number, the more effective, although a 30 sunscreen is only about 5 percent more effective than a 15. And keep in mind, a 15 SPF on the *skin* is better than a 30 SPF in the *bottle*." Sun exposure can also increase the likelihood of cataracts, so wear sunglasses with UV protection. I took his advice several years ago and started wearing a tightly woven hat with a brim, along with my daily applications of sunscreen.

Suspicious Moles

What do you do if you find a mole that is growing, or has flaky, itchy skin and doesn't heal? Go to a dermatologist and have it checked.

Sunburn Home Remedy

Dr. Lynch recommends aspirin dissolved in water and applied to the skin as the best emergency first-aid treatment for sunburn. If you're on a camping trip, get a burn, and don't have a bottle of aloe vera gel (or before you put on the aloe vera), use the aspirin-water application. "Aspirin orally is effective, along with the topical aspirin, and cold compresses are also helpful," Dr. Lynch concluded. Use 1-2 aspirin tablets dissolved in ¼ cup of water.

Skin spots, which can turn into precancerous lesions or even skin cancer if left too long, are easy enough to take care of. So don't wait, expecting the spot to heal on its own. Most dermatologists use cryosurgery, a simple procedure of freezing the spot with liquid nitrogen. The sooner you have it checked, the easier it is to cure.

Body Odor

No doubt about it, if you exercise in any form, you're going to sweat. It's a natural part of being human, a way the body cleanses the skin and gets rid of toxic waste. The act of sweating isn't what causes odor; it's the bacteria that grow as a result of the moisture.

Men have more, and larger, sweat glands than do women. Probably back when we all lived in caves, we found each other by smell, much as wild animals still do. It's been proven that pheromones, natural chemical attractants found in sweat and body odor, play a role in how we are attracted to each other.

Many years ago, when I was in the landscaping business, I had several college students working for me. On one particular job, three of us were riding in the company truck every day for several months. The trip took more than a half hour, the weather was hot, the work dirty. Both of the workers on that crew came to work daily wearing only shoes and gym shorts. One of the guys, Dan, was a long-haired hippie college student, by his own description. Bob, the other fellow, was a college jock and lived in a dorm. He always smelled newly washed, like soap. But when Dan got in the truck, it almost made our eyes water. His body odor was so bad that finally one day Bob just asked him, "Dan, do you realize that you smell worse when you come to work in the morning than I do at the end of the day?"

"Yeah," Dan said with a sly grin. "My old lady really digs how I smell. It turns her on and we copulate like monkeys when I get home from work. I don't want to ruin that." Bob and I quickly realized that we weren't going to talk Dan into better hygiene if good sex with his girlfriend was the payoff. We just started making Dan sit next to the window, and asked that he keep his pits covered with his arms. Other than Dan's girlfriend, I've never heard of another woman turned on by raunchy body odor. However, movie star Brad Pitt has a reputation for liking the reek of his own sweat, and plenty of women are excited by him, so perhaps I'm wrong.

Bathe too often and you get itchy skin; bathe too seldom and people stand at a distance, sniffing the air and making faces. What's a guy to do? I think finding a happy medium, of not being overly perfumed but not reeking of soggy underarms, might be the better choice.

Combating Body Odor with Herbs

Sweat is caused by secretions from apocrine sweat glands, which are found primarily under the arms. Bacteria grow in the secretions and odor develops, not from the sweat, but from the bacteria that thrive in the moisture. Males start developing body odor during puberty.

Several problems contribute to excessive body odor. A zinc deficiency can encourage body odor, as can just plain poor hygiene. Odor can also be a result of diabetes, liver problems, chronic constipation, and even diet. The times I've tried being mostly vegetarian, I've noticed that my red-meat-eating friends smell different, and my staunchly vegetarian friends tell me that they can always tell just by standing next to someone whether that person is a meat-eater; to them, meat-eaters definitely smell different. If you have a problem with chronic body odor, be sure to visit your doctor to rule out an ailment.

There are several herbs that combat body odor or are useful as deodorants. Herbs that have an antibacterial action are the most effective. Coriander and licorice both have a high number of antibacterial chemicals, as do oregano, rosemary, and ginger. Thyme has excellent antibacterial action and I use it in several of my soaking bath blends. You'll even find thymol, or oil of thyme, listed as an antibacterial ingredient in Listerine mouthwash. Lavender oil, also, is antibacterial.

Using Diet to Correct Odor

Medical anthropologist John Heinerman, Ph.D., says in his book *Heinerman's Encyclopedia of Fruits, Vegetables, and Herbs* that turnips help prevent body odor. He buzzed up some raw turnips in his juicer, then applied a teaspoonful under each arm. "Turnip juice won't prevent sweating, but it keeps body odor from occurring for about 10 hours," he said. Probably not many guys would be willing to slather turnip juice under their arms, but there's the information if you're bored and want to check it out.

Probably a better thing to do is to eat plenty of vegetables that contain zinc, or even take zinc supplements if odor is a big problem. (Really bad foot odor often responds well to an increase in zinc in the diet, also). Good sources of zinc include:

- Spinach
- Collard greens
- Brussels sprouts
- Parsley
- Cucumbers
- String beans
- Prunes
- Asparagus
- Endive

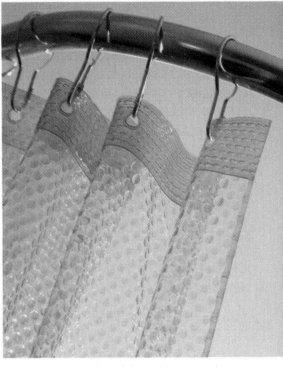

A daily shower or bath followed by a good deodorant will help keep you smelling clean. Look to dietary modifications if body odor is a chronic problem.

But this list is generally what most guys try to *avoid* eating. Parsley is good, especially the flat-leafed Italian variety, but the rest I can pretty well do without. If you feel the same, consider adding a zinc supplement to your diet and see if it doesn't help fight body odor.

→ Garlic, Valerian, and Skin Scent

Eating lots of garlic or taking valerian capsules (an herb used for relaxing muscles) can change a man's body odor. We secrete moisture through the skin, and if the moisture contains something pungent, like garlic oil, the skin will smell like a bit of the same thing. What you eat in quantity can make your skin taste different to your sex partner, as well.

Using Homemade Deodorants

Why, you might wonder, would anyone want to make something that is so easy to buy? First, lots of deodorants can clog up the natural breathing and sweating process of the skin. Some deodorants actually have ingredients that close up the sweat cells, which can lead to infection, rashes, and soreness. Or maybe you're allergic to the chemicals. Perhaps you'd just like an easy alternative. These formulas are meant for soaking up moisture and thus preventing bacteria from growing, rather than adding a perfume that only masks the odor of sweat.

Herbal Underarm Solution

John Heinerman, Ph.D., says that vinegar is another effective underarm deodorant. Vinegar prevents the growth of bacteria and, thus, the odor. However, I doubt that many of us really want to walk around smelling like a pickle. Here's a method that utilizes the effectiveness of vinegar but has a more pleasant smell. Use dried herbs in this formula.

> 2½ cups white or cider vinegar
> 2 tablespoons shavegrass (*Equisetum hyemale* —
>   don't substitute another variety!)
> 1 tablespoon lemongrass
> 1 tablespoon ground or chopped sage
> 1 teaspoon thyme
> 1 teaspoon lavender
> ½ teaspoon mint
> ¼ cup bottled water

1. In a saucepan, bring the vinegar almost to boiling. Add the remaining ingredients, including the water, and let steep, covered, overnight.

2. Strain, discarding the solids, and bottle the liquid. Store in a cool, dark place.

3. To use, soak a corner of a washcloth with the liquid and wipe under the arms. If this burns or feels too strong, cut it with another ¼ cup of water.

Underarm B.O. Absorber

Baking soda and cornstarch are helpful as an underarm deodorant (and for an in-the-socks dust). A 50-50 mixture is drying, discourages bacterial growth (because of the drier conditions), and absorbs odor. If you're allergic to underarm deodorants, this is an easy-to-make alternative. And, even better, it's cheap.

> 1 cup cornstarch
> ½ cup baking soda (not baking powder —
> there's a difference!)
> 6 drops bay rum essential oil
> 2 drops clove essential oil

1. Put everything in a food processor (or mix in a bowl by hand). Pulse several times, then pour into a container with a shaker lid, such as a kitchen salt shaker.

2. Shake out a small amount in the palm of your hand and apply it to the underarms. Pat the area just enough to spread the dust around but not leave big clumps. This is also fine to use in the groin area to absorb moisture. Use after bathing.

Camper's Quick Fixes

In *The Herbal Home Spa* (Storey Books, 1998), Greta Breedlove suggests a lemon as an underarm deodorant. In a pinch, like on a camping trip, it's worth a try. Lemon juice is too acidic for bacteria to grow. She suggests cutting a lemon in half and rubbing it under your arms. The next time you've forgotten your deodorant and have a fresh lemon handy, check it out. Watch out, though, or you'll be known as "ol' lemon pits" in the workout room.

If you're on a trip in the great outdoors and can't bathe, use moist towelettes, such as unscented baby wipes, to wash underarms, feet, and groin, then apply the Underarm B.O. Absorber dust. It will leave you feeling like you've had a bath, and everyone around you will appreciate the effort.

The Dreaded Warts

Most people don't like to talk about warts. They're kind of disgusting, show up without obvious reason, and are hard to remove.

There are all kinds of folk remedies for warts, many dating back to the 17th and 18th centuries in England, even though we may think of the remedies as purely American. Like the one my friend Mikul told me from his family: "You have to steal your grandmother's dishrag without her knowing. Wipe it over the wart, then bury the rag in your backyard," he said.

Another old folk remedy, which seems to be purely Ozark in origin, calls for you to catch a grasshopper and hold the insect up to the wart. "The grasshopper will start nibbling on the wart and it doesn't grow back," says Tina Marie Wilcox, head gardener and folk historian at the Heritage Herb Garden at the Ozark Folk Center State Park in Arkansas.

Old herbals claim that cutting a houseleek (*Sempervivum* sp., a common rock-garden plant also known as hens and chicks) leaf in half and squeezing out the slippery liquid on the wart every day is a cure. I've heard friends swear that this method worked for them. They cut the leaf in half and place the sticky side on the wart, then cover with an adhesive bandage.

Warts are unpredictable, and can go away as mysteriously as they appeared. There is a tradition in some communities of a wart-removing person. The one I knew was a woman in Texas. She told me that the knowledge was passed on to her from her father, and she could pass it along only to her son, not to a daughter. Lots of very happy people in that community claimed they had their warts removed magically by this woman.

Conventional Therapies

So what really works and what doesn't? There are scores of different home remedies, and if your luck holds, one may seem to work just because the wart is likely to leave on its own (even though it may come back).

Warts are caused by HPV, the human papillomavirus, a very common virus with about 60 variations. One kind of HPV causes genital warts, another causes warts on the hands, and so on. Here's a rundown of more predictable treatments:

Over-the-counter preparations to remove warts such as Compound W and DuoFilm contain salicylic acid and basically dissolve small warts. The product is to be applied daily for about a month and the wart should fall off. Dr. Terrence Cronin, who is a dermatologist at the University of Miami, warns "Skin cancer sometimes looks like a wart; [therefore,] if the wart doesn't respond to salicylic acid after four weeks, let a dermatologist inspect the site."

Surgery, a more serious kind of wart removal, can be done on an out-patient basis by a dermatologist. Cryotherapy is the most likely method the doctor will use, and it consists of freezing the wart with liquid nitrogen. There's very little pain involved, mostly a slight swelling and irritation for a day after the procedure, and within a week or 10 days the wart will shrivel and fall off. Cryotherapy, also called cryosurgery, costs $80 to $100 and takes but minutes to perform.

Laser surgery is another option, although the cost for this starts at more than $100 and generally runs closer to $500 per visit. Carbon dioxide lasers scorch the wart and pulse-dye lasers work on the blood vessels that feed the wart area. The wart will shrivel in a few weeks.

There are also newer treatments on the horizon for genital warts. Two recent drugs, Condylox and Aldara, are showing real promise in this area. Consult your dermatologist if this is your problem.

Herbal Remedies That *Really* Work

Terry Willard, a medical herbalist, claims, "By far, my favorite remedy for warts is the fresh white latex from dandelion stems." He suggests picking a dandelion flower stem and covering the entire wart with the juice that oozes from the stem. "This has to be continued three times a day for 7 to 10 days. The wart will turn black and fall off. I've been recommending this technique to my patients for some 20 years, and it's more than 80 percent effective," Willard said.

If dandelions aren't in season or available, he suggests blackened banana peels. Apply the inside of the peel to the wart, keeping a small piece in place with an adhesive strip for 6 to 8 hours each day for 10 days. And, says Willard, "Thuja oil applied externally is also quite effective."

The Herb Pharm, a manufacturer of medicinal tinctures, recommends a blend in liquid extract of lomatium root *(Lomatium dissectum)*, St. John's wort *(Hypericum perforatum)*, hyssop *(Hyssopus officinalis)*, lemon balm *(Melissa officinalis)*, thuja *(Thuja occidentalis)*, and echinacea seed *(Echinacea purpurea)*. See Resources for contact information for the Herb Pharm.

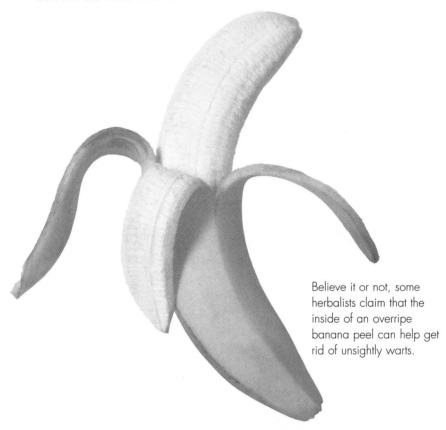

Believe it or not, some herbalists claim that the inside of an overripe banana peel can help get rid of unsightly warts.

→ What Not to Do

Don't use the time-honored "real man's" remedy and chisel away at the wart with your pocketknife. While this may make you feel like you're accomplishing something by taking action, you're actually spreading the virus through the small tissue fragments you whittle off, which reinfect surrounding skin. Doing this increases the likelihood that the wart will spread.

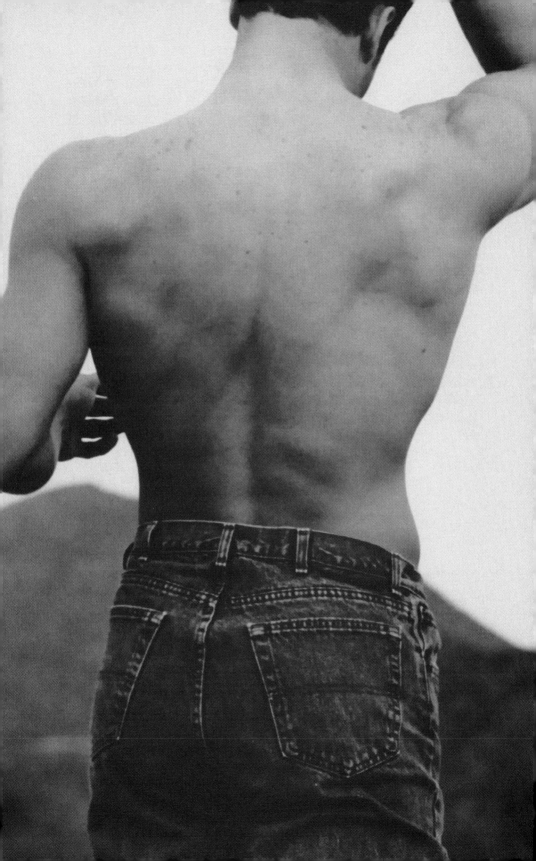

Chapter 4
below the belt

■ THE SKY DIVERS

For about 20 years I was in the nursery business, and at one point had as employees two sky divers. Ted, who was 25, and Sarah, who was 35, lived together in an honest-to-goodness tepee in the woods. Both were avid career sky divers, having met on a jump over a remote stretch of desert in New Mexico a couple of years before.

The two of them built their tepee deep in the Ozark woods on a 1,200-acre piece of land that was mostly untouched by modern development. Giant pines, remnants of the trees that once covered large sections of the Ozarks, stood on ridge tops that were inaccessible to loggers when the surrounding land was cleared, around the turn of the century, for railroad ties. The pair had the guts to do what few other people ever do: They followed their dreams.

Ted and Sarah cooked on a campfire, including baking their bread. They even made pies in a crude oven. They grew an admirable garden, filled with vegetables, flowers, and herbs, and they dried the vegetables, used the herbs in cooking and healing, and worked toward being self-sufficient. They bathed daily, winter and summer, in a crystal-clear stream beside the tepee, and carried their drinking water from a nearby spring that bubbled pure and cold out of a limestone bluff.

Both of these folks had always been city dwellers. Ted grew up in a densely populated part of downtown San Francisco, an area he referred to as "just a ghetto," while Sarah was raised in the Chicago suburbs. Both took to sky diving like they had been born to it, and I used to read about their record-setting achievements in the sports pages of magazines. Once they set the record for the largest number of divers to link up while sky diving naked, and the magazine article showed a very distant photo of 17 or so naked-as-jaybirds divers holding hands in the sky as they fell 10,000 feet a second (or whatever that speed is when an object falls).

"What'd it feel like, Ted?" I asked one day as we ate lunch at the nursery, a bunch of workers sitting around idly chatting.

"Oh, imagine your testicles packed in ice, a 200-mile-an-hour wind blowing up your butt, air rushing at you so fast that it's flattening out your face like a pie hitting a wall, while you're falling at 300 feet a second," he answered. "All the time you're determined to ignore every human instinct for the sole purpose of joining hands with a bunch of really crazy folks seconds before you crash to the ground and become just another bug splat on the pavement. It was awesome!" he finished with a huge grin and a chuckle.

Sometimes they'd do jumps into a mall parking lot for pay. It was always a grand opening for a new store or theater, and there'd be a bull's-eye target about 20 feet across on the pavement. Ted said hitting the target was easy, even from thousands of feet in the air, but hitting the pavement could be tricky. "You don't want to do it if you've got back problems," he said to me one day. "And slamming into asphalt at that speed too often, if you're fighting a crosswind, can be hard on both your teeth and your prostate if you don't judge the fall just right. We all carry a bottle of aspirin with us," he concluded, "and a pint of Jim Beam."

Watching the couple was fascinating for everyone at the nursery. Ted, trying to be the dominant male provider, was always surprising Sarah with little presents to make her life easier. He once bought her, as a Christmas gift, a liner for their tepee. "It's insulation, a liner with an air space," Ted told me when I asked about it. "One more layer against blowing snow this winter."

Out of the blue Ted would buy Sarah a cooking pan, or find a new kind of tea, or a book. Sarah told me quietly one day when Ted was away at one of our landscape jobs, "He's so sweet, but he just doesn't get it. I don't want to be a housewife. If I did, I sure wouldn't be sleeping on the ground in a tepee!"

The couple seemed to navigate gingerly the deep waters of compromise and had the kind of relationship that many couples only wish they had. Ted was young, full of energy, exciting, and very sexual. Sarah had been married to a vanilla-in-the-suburbs kind of guy. She had tried that and didn't like the experience. "No," she said. "When I was married, there was no excitement. With Ted, every day is an adventure. Imagine, we've been on our honeymoon for more than two years and the new still hasn't worn off!"

One chilly morning in early April, the pair appeared at work late, both looking like they had been caught beneath an 18-wheeler and dragged for miles. "What on earth happened to you two?" I inquired. "Flood," was all Ted would say. He was slamming doors and in a foul mood.

As the story came out, Sarah described how the pair had gone to sleep under a partly cloudy spring sky. During the night it began to rain. They both stirred but went back to sleep. "By about, oh, I don't know, maybe 3 A.M., I woke up with water under my sleeping bag. I nudged Ted and he grunted and rolled over and went back to sleep," Sarah said.

But the water got deeper and Ted finally got up. He found flashlights and launched himself out the tepee's door. "He was swearing like a Marine," Sarah said, half laughing, half still overwhelmed by the experience. "If you take out all the swearing," she continued, "what you'd have left is, 'There's an awful lot of water out here.' "

It seems the placid little stream that was so romantic when they first placed the tepee on the bank had risen during the night, filling to overflowing by the hard rains. The creek had risen more than 5 feet, washing away the dishes they'd left in the water after dinner. Their garden tools had been swept downstream, along with all the 5-gallon buckets that they used to carry water.

In total darkness, water around their feet and rising several inches a minute, they had gathered up everything they could find — sleeping bags, clothing, food, radios, lanterns, guitar — and carried it all through the woods to higher ground, throwing everything into a soggy pile in the still-driving, chilly rain. When they arrived at work, they had already spent several hours salvaging their belongings and were wet, cold, and exhausted. I told them to go home and repair what they could, and after work several of us went over to help.

Luckily, the next several days were sunny. The stream fell as quickly as it had risen, and the tepee wasn't seriously damaged. It leaned a little, from the current of the water, the long poles that held open the smoke flap were askew, but otherwise the structure was in pretty good shape. Ted righted the tepee, they dried out their sleeping bags in a laundromat, and over the next few weeks found most of their tools and dishes about a quarter of a mile downstream, caught up in a driftwood dam the flood had left.

"So does this mean you'll be moving the tepee to higher ground?" I asked Ted. "Oh, no. We like where it is. One flood out of two years isn't bad. We'll just be sure to have better flashlight batteries from now on," he said with a laugh and a wave of his hand.

Many men go through early life not thinking much about the health of the area below the belt. But whether we like it or not, as we age, we eventually have to consider how to keep the prostate healthy and how to keep our more private body parts in good working order. Following are useful herbal preparations, tips, and suggestions for keeping those areas healthy.

The Prostate

There are lots of things that can cause prostate problems. Falls out of airplanes onto pavement, like Ted used to do, can jar you all over. But lots of other accidents can contribute to problems, as well.

I once fell on the ice, one of those tumbles where you're on the ground before your mind realizes it should have reminded you to throw out a hand to break the fall. My feet flew out from under me and I landed flat on my butt. By the next day I had a lot of pain in my prostate. When I went to the doctor he said, "Oh, surely it can't be your prostate. How do you even know where your prostate is, anyway?" I assured him that I did know where my body parts are, and that I did, indeed, know how a bruised prostate felt. He suggested aspirin and obviously didn't believe I knew what I'd bruised. I soaked myself in a hot herbal bath, took aspirin, and in a few days I was feeling better. Sore, but better.

The Dangers of Too Much Sitting

Of all the things men have to look out for to avoid damage to the prostate gland, one of the worst is sitting. If you have a job where you sit for long stretches, eventually you're likely to have prostate problems. These problems are caused by pressure on and lack of circulation to the prostate.

7Song, an herbal practitioner in Ithaca, New York, says that you should get up and move or exercise every 15 or 20 minutes if you have a desk job. "Lots of men will sit at their desk for two, three, or more hours without ever moving," he says. "Then they wonder why they can't sleep at night, because their prostate is hurting. That problem is easily avoided by exercise. Get up and move around, dance, walk, anything to keep up the circulation," he suggests.

Caring for the Prostate through Diet

Mickey Spillane said, "If you don't take care of your body, where are you going to live?"

So how does a guy take care of his prostate? Exercise and diet are at the top of the list, along with a healthy sex life; there is some evidence that men who have sex regularly are less likely to have prostate problems later than men who have sex infrequently.

A study from the American Cancer Society followed 480,000 men for a dozen years to see if there was a correlation between women who have breast cancer and their sons' risk of prostate cancer. Men who had three or more close female relatives who had breast cancer had a 63 percent greater risk of dying from prostate cancer. The study showed that men under 50 were at greatest risk. But Carmen Rodriguez, M.D., who led the study, said, "Certain things are risk factors for both prostate and breast cancer, such as a high fat intake." It's just another indication that the kind of food you eat does affect your health, or lack of it.

Researchers at the East Carolina University School of Medicine, in studies led by Manfred Steiner, M.D., found that a chemical (S-allylmercapto-cysteine, or SAMC) killed prostate cancer cells in laboratory experiments. Garlic powders and oils contain a little SAMC, but fresh garlic and aged garlic supplements both contain more SAMC. Other research, including studies by the National Cancer Institute, has shown that fresh fruits and vegetables lower the risk of many kinds of cancer. They suggest that you can have a 70 percent lower risk of cancer if you make sure to eat plenty of fruits and vegetables (five servings a day). An easy way to ensure that you get the recommended amount is never to eat a meal that doesn't include at least one fruit or vegetable and to drink fruit juice instead of a soft drink.

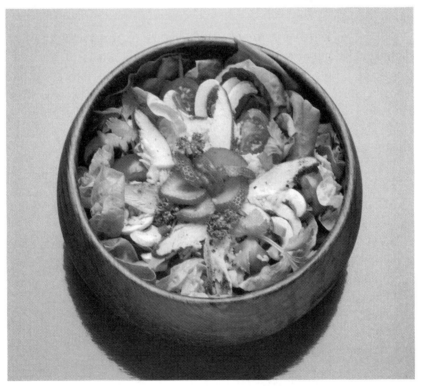

You probably won't be surprised to hear that diet is the best way to influence prostate health. So what are you waiting for?

Extra-Healthy Tuna Salad Sandwich

Here's an easy way to get a couple of small servings of fresh vegetables for lunch. This is a very tasty, low-fat, high-in-vegetables sandwich. Tuna is touted as a healthy food, one more reason to like this meal. I learned to make this from my friend Josh years ago, and he learned to make it from a friend who ran a vegetarian restaurant (don't groan, this isn't your mom's tuna salad but a hearty, healthy sandwich), and guests at my house often ask for the recipe. Watch your coworkers scarf down a burger and fries while you think to yourself how healthy this lunch is.

2 pillows plain shredded wheat
(large pillows, not bite-sized)
2 cans (6 ounces each) tuna, packed in water
2 tablespoons chopped sweet pickles
½ cup low-fat mayonnaise
2 stalks celery, cut into chunks
1 slice onion
2 carrots, peeled and cut into chunks
Pinch of caraway seed (what you can pinch
between your thumb and forefinger)

1. In a mixing bowl, crush the shredded wheat. Open the tuna and drain out most of the water. Add the tuna, sweet pickles, and mayonnaise to the crushed wheat, and stir. Set aside.

2. In a food processor (or use a hand grater), grate the celery, onion, and carrots with the caraway seed. Add that to the tuna mix and blend well. Add a bit more mayonnaise if needed; you want it moist enough to stick together but not drenched. Mix again and refrigerate. (This will keep about a week in the refrigerator, although it seldom lasts that long at my house because we eat it so quickly.)

3. Spread the tuna salad generously on whole-grain or multigrain bread, top with lettuce, and finish with a second slice of bread. If you add an apple to your lunch, you get grains, vegetables, protein (tuna), fruit, and fiber, all of which are believed to be good for lowering cholesterol and keeping the colon and prostate healthy.

Prostate First Aid and Maintenance

7Song is the director of the Northeast School of Botanical Medicine in Ithaca, New York. A respected teacher and lecturer on men's health issues, he agreed to share his prostate herbal treatments. These are his formulas, made from herbs that have earned a reputation for helping with problems of the prostate.

Prostate Tonic Tincture

This tincture is useful for easing pain in the prostate and the resulting difficulty with urination, as well as maintaining the health of the prostate.

> 3 tablespoons whole saw palmetto
> berries (Serenoa repens)
> 2 tablespoons nettles, leaf and root (Urtica spp.)
> 2 teaspoons echinacea root (Echinacea spp.)
> 2 teaspoons corn silk (Zea mays)
> 2 teaspoons couch grass (Agropyron repens)
> 2 teaspoons marsh mallow root (Althea officinalis)
> 2 cups vodka
> ½ cup bottled or distilled water

1. Combine the herbs and vodka in a glass or plastic container with a tight lid. Shake the container and set aside, shaking daily for 15 days.
2. Strain out and discard the herbs. Add the bottled or distilled water to the liquid.
3. To use for severe pain or difficulty urinating, 7Song recommends 1 teaspoon in half a glass of water or juice two or three times daily, being sure to stop at least 2 hours before bedtime. The maintenance dose is 1 teaspoon in a half glass of water or juice every other day.

Take Care with Calcium

Calcium is necessary for the maintenance of bones and teeth, as we know. But you can take in too much calcium, according to Peter D. Fugelso, M.D., the medical director of the Kidney Stone Department at St. Joseph's Medical Center in Burbank, California. He says, "If you are taking supplements with calcium, the first thing to do is check with your doctor to see if they are really necessary." He says that for people who have, or had, kidney stones, too much calcium can make fertile ground for more stones. If kidney stones are a concern, he suggests you not take antacids that are calcium-based and not partake heavily of oxalate-rich foods. Those include chocolate, grapes, green peppers, parsley, spinach, summer squash, beets, blueberries, and celery. (He doesn't say you should eliminate them, just cut back.)

Prostate Tea

Make up using all dried herbs, then take out the amount you need when you want to make tea. The same herbs are used in both parts of this formula, but the decoction contains roots and berries while the infusion contains the leaves and flowers. It sounds complicated, but a simple method for making the tea follows. 7Song says this drink is effective against prostate infection and difficulty with urination.

Note: *7Song cautions that if you have high blood pressure or are taking a diuretic for blood pressure, the licorice should be left out of the recipe. In some people, licorice can cause increased sodium retention.*

Part 1

1 tablespoon couch grass rhizome (*Agropyron repens*)

3 tablespoons dandelion root (*Taraxacum officinale*)

1 tablespoon gravelroot (*Eupatorium purpureum*)

½ teaspoon licorice root (*Glycyrrhiza glabra*)

1 tablespoon stoneroot (*Collinsonia canadensis*)

2 tablespoons saw palmetto berries (cut and sifted, or broken berries) (*Serenoa repens*)

1 teaspoon echinacea root (*Echinacea* spp.)

Large pinch of goldenseal (*Hydrastis canadensis*), cut and sifted (root is preferred, but if all you can find is the ground herb, use slightly less than ⅛ teaspoon)

Part 2

4 tablespoons raspberry leaves (*Rubus idaeus*)

4 tablespoons nettle leaves (*Urtica* spp.)

2 tablespoons oatstraw (*Avena sativa*)

1 tablespoon echinacea leaves and flowers (*Echinacea* spp.)

2 tablespoons dandelion leaves (*Taraxacum officinale*)

1 teaspoon parsley leaves (*Petroselinum crispum*)

1¼ teaspoons marsh mallow leaves (*Althea officinalis*)

½ teaspoon yarrow leaves and flower (*Achillea millefolium*)

1. In a mixing bowl, combine all the herbs in Part 1. Place in a zipper-lock bag and set aside.

2. Combine all the herbs in Part 2. Place in a separate plastic zipper-lock bag or container and set aside.

3. Mix or stir *each bag* of herbs separately before taking any out. This is important because some parts have a tendency to settle to the bottom.

4. Bring 6 cups of water to a boil and add ½ cup of the just stirred Part 1 mix. Lower the heat, and let the mixture simmer, covered, for 20 minutes.

5. Turn off the heat. Immediately add ½ cup of the Part 2 mix and stir into the liquid. Let steep, covered, for 10 minutes.

6. Strain. Drink an 8-ounce glass of the tea in the morning and again in the afternoon. Or put a glassful on your desk and sip it during the day. The tea should be at room temperature or warm when drunk; cold drinks can aggravate the prostate. Refrigerate any leftovers. Stop drinking the tea 4 hours before going to bed; otherwise you'll be getting up to pee during the night.

Saw Palmetto and Prostate Health

Saw palmetto *(Serenoa repens)* is a shrublike palm that grows in the southeastern United States. Saw palmetto sales account for about $25 million of Florida's annual economy, according to Ted Helms of the state agriculture department.

Saw palmetto is used primarily in the treatment of benign prostatic hyperplasia (BPH), enlargement of the prostate gland. Fifty percent of men over 50 suffer from this ailment, four out of five men over 80 are afflicted, and even some men in their 40s are affected. In combination with pumpkin seed and stinging nettle root, it is believed to help regulate hormone metabolism. Medical studies in Germany, France, and elsewhere have demonstrated that BPH responds well to treatments of saw palmetto, minimizing swelling and frequent nighttime urination.

Steven Foster, author of nine books on herbal health, cautions, "While much of the news about saw palmetto is good, some medical practitioners say they are concerned that its use could be risky: The symptoms of BPH and prostate cancer are similar, so using palmetto . . . may simultaneously relieve symptoms and mask signs of a more serious nature. Therefore, say medical practitioners, stay in touch with your health-care provider and don't bypass regular screening for prostate cancer."

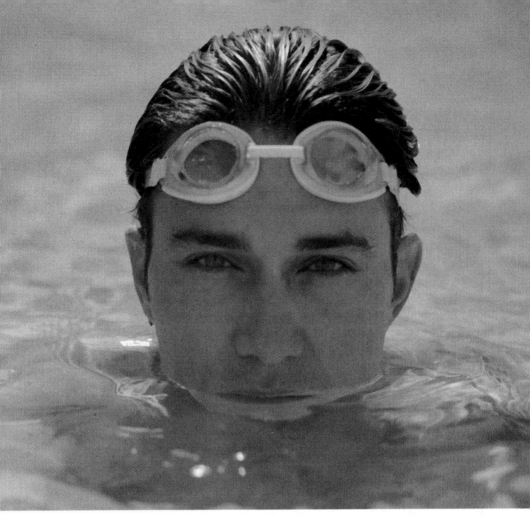

Stay active to keep your body in the best condition possible. You can choose from a variety of activities to keep your routine interesting.

Stress, Red Green, Duct Tape, and Sheer Manliness

Dr. Ira Sharlip, professor of urology at the University of California, San Francisco, contends that relaxing the body's muscles helps in the treatment of chronic, nonbacterial prostatitis. He says that stress, and the accompanying muscle tension, is one cause of men's prostate problems. 7Song recommends dance, sports, exercise, and other types of movement to reduce stress. Play golf, swim, walk, run, whatever it takes to relax. Then, when you're really tired and ready to sit again, have ready a stress-reducing distraction. I'll share with you one of my favorite books for reading in short spurts to relax, and I'll also tell you about my favorite man's TV show.

Check out *The Big Damn Book of Sheer Manliness,* by Todd and Brandt von Hoffman. In it, you will discover the origin of the tommy gun, learn 256 names for a man's sex organ, and find out about the "mud flap Girl" (you know, the reclining naked lady on the mud flaps of 18-wheelers). The book also gives championship chili cook-offs and barbecues as destinations for really manly outings. You'll find the origin of WD-40, and lots of information about the many uses of duct tape. If you want more stress-reducing information about duct tape, go to the Duct Tape Page on the Internet (see Resources for address). You'll laugh (and after all, that's part of reducing stress).

Another site that isn't all duct tape but purportedly boosted duct tape sales nationwide through his very popular television show is www. redgreen.com. Red Green is the star (and the name) of the all-man show. Red builds cool stuff from duct tape (of course it never works, which is part of the comedy). The first time you watch the show, be prepared to think it's strange. The next time you watch, you'll probably begin to identify it as "pure man stuff" and plenty of fun. I've met very few women who can watch the show all the way through.

I went to an appearance of Red Green a year ago at our local PBS station. I knew it would be crowded, so I arrived an hour late. When I got there, people were standing in a line four bodies wide, stretching for a block and a half. Those folks had been there for more than two hours just to catch a glimpse of Red. I waited for almost that long, the line barely moving (this was a Junior League event, handled by volunteers who'd brought a little bowl of cookies and a coffeepot, never realizing that hundreds of working men would arrive). Finally, they trotted Red down the line to shake hands with everyone in the very tired but certainly eager crowd.

The best part, though, was seeing who his fans are. Out of maybe 800 or 1,000 people, 90 percent were men and children and 50 percent or more had their own rolls of duct tape in hand, on their wrist, taped to their belts, or hanging from their tool belts. If you haven't discovered the *Red Green Show,* from Canada, by and for men, you're in for a real treat. Check the Web site to find a public television station near you that carries it. I'm convinced that doctors could write a prescription to their stressed-out patients to watch Red Green, and see positive results in less than two weeks!

Truck drivers who travel long distances without taking a break or moving also experience varying kinds of prostate problems. Whether you're a long-distance driver or a desk worker, if there's no choice about frequent breaks or changing positions, butt-clench exercises can help to keep the circulation going. Simply flex the buttocks while you sit, like you're trying to crack a walnut between your butt cheeks. Flex 10 to 20 times every half hour or so. Getting up and stretching, walking, or bending over and touching your toes is helpful also. Taking frequent breaks from a static position is essential for the prostate, as well as to help keep up circulation.

Penile Drip

Ever wonder why old men smell like, well, old men? There can be more than one reason, but the primary one is that lots of men in old age (four out of five men over the age of 80) suffer from prostate problems, which can cause improper shutoff of their urine flow. Throughout the day a little dribble here, a little dribble there, and soon the old guy's smelling like he's peed his pants. (Combine that with a man's decrease in his sense of smell as he ages, and the fact that lots of older men think that because they haven't done any physical labor all day, or all week, those same clothes should be good for several days in a row, and you have an old fellow who smells like an old man, can't smell himself, and doesn't want to change clothes — all in all, pretty frustrating for those around him.)

Keeping the prostate healthy is important to avoid this problem. If you're dealing with your father or grandfather, you may have to tactfully and carefully tell him that he probably doesn't realize it, but he stinks. After all, your father probably changed your diapers and showed concern for your urinary habits when you were a baby. As your father ages, you may have to return the favor. It's just part of the cycle of life, neither pleasant nor awful, just a fact.

More Tips for Prostate Health

James Duke, in *The Green Pharmacy,* says that ginkgo promotes blood flow to the brain. "But it also seems to boost blood flow into the penis, thus aiding iffy erections," he said. He quotes several studies that have shown excellent results using ginkgo to treat impotence due to atherosclerotic clogging of the penile artery.

James Green, in *The Male Herbal,* suggests several things a man can do to help his prostate when he's having pain or irritation:

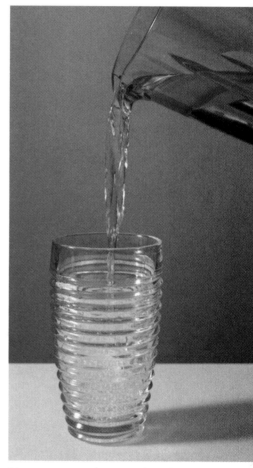

- Relax, using herbs like valerian, crampbark, and skullcap (all good muscle-relaxers) when needed.
- Drink plenty of water and avoid large amounts of cold beer (cold seems to make prostate problems worse, according to several authorities).
- Eat a diet high in whole grains, a variety of fresh or steamed vegetables, and fruit.
- Eat seeds, like pumpkin, poppy, sunflower, and sesame (available in health-food stores); pumpkin seeds, especially, are important for a healthy prostate, and Green recommends eating a half cup of the hulled seeds daily.
- Take vitamin and mineral supplements, such as 800 IU of vitamin E, 400 to 600 mg calcium/magnesium combination, and 20 to 50 mg zinc picolinate or amino chelated zinc.

Additionally, Green recommends hot and cold packs applied to the skin surrounding the prostate area (between the scrotum and the anus) to reduce inflammation and swelling of the

How many times have you heard that you should drink lots of water? It's true: Drinking eight or more glasses a day is recommended for urinary and prostate health.

prostate. Apply a hot pack, such as a damp washcloth, for about 5 minutes and immediately follow that with ice wrapped in a cloth for 1 to 2 minutes. Repeat the entire process. Following this hot-cold routine a couple of times a day, says Green, will reduce the inflammation and bring relief to a swollen prostate (this method also works for other swollen body parts).

Note: A clean sock makes a pretty good ice pack. Just throw half a dozen ice cubes into a dampened sock. Or use a zipper-lock sandwich bag to hold the ice cubes inside the damp sock.

Treating Urinary Tract Infections

Urinary tract infections are much less common in men than in women, but men occasionally contract infections that cause painful inflammation of the tube leading from the bladder to the tip of the penis. Be sure to visit your doctor right away if you experience pain or burning during urination, or difficulty in urinating. Blood in the urine, while usually a sign of a more serious problem, can sometimes be the result of a urinary tract infection.

There are several ways to reduce your risk of contracting a urinary tract infection. Drinking lots of water and urinating frequently is the most recommended method. Maureen Sangiorgio, in the December 1998 issue of *Reader's Digest,* suggests that urinary tract infections respond quickly to cranberry juice. She quotes Dr. Mari-Kim Brunnell, an OB/GYN at Brigham and Women's Hospital in Boston, as saying, "Cranberry juice prevents bacteria from sticking to the lining of the urinary tract." A study reported in the *Journal of the American Medical Association* recommends drinking 10 ounces of cranberry juice daily if you are prone to urinary infections. If you're bothered by the acid, cut the juice by half with water, but drink the full amount of juice that's recommended.

Cranberry-Yogurt Drink

My method for keeping the urinary tract healthy is to combine active-culture yogurt with cranberry juice. The yogurt seems to make the acid more digestible. If you're not crazy about the taste of cranberry juice, the honey will sweeten it and make it more palatable.

> 8 to 10 ounces pure cranberry juice (check the label:
> Some bottled juices have only 15 or
> 20 percent juice)
> ¼ cup plain low-fat yogurt
> 2 teaspoons honey (optional)

Combine the juice, yogurt, and the honey, if desired, in a blender and pulse-blend until smooth. Drink a glass of the mixture with breakfast two or three times a week to maintain a healthy urinary tract. When you have an infection, Dr. Brunnell suggests using the full 10 ounces of cranberry juice. Drink it frequently throughout the day.

Aphrodisiacs

Many herbs have been considered aphrodisiacs throughout history. Some are still in use today. Certain vegetables, those that have some vague resemblance to the male sex organ, have also had some reputation for that purpose. An example is asparagus. Because it looks like the erect male member, it was considered an aphrodisiac. And probably because it made urine stink in many men, it was believed to be powerful and useful. (Did you know that not every man's urine smells after eating asparagus? It's supposedly related to body chemistry, but it's one of the main reasons that men often say they don't like asparagus.) While there are plenty of supposed aphrodisiacs that don't really work, there are also several herbs and foods that have garnered a deserved reputation for aiding the libido.

Herbs for Love?

Here are several herbs that were used in past centuries for curing impotence or awakening lust, or both:

Clary sage *(Salvia sclarea).* Gerard, an early herbalist and researcher writing in the 1600s, thought that clary sage had some merit as an aphrodisiac: "The seed poudered and drunke with wine, stirreth up bodily lust." There seems to be no proof of its usefulness as an aphrodisiac, however, but you can experiment by using a chopped-up, fresh clary sage leaf in a mixture of red wine and lemon, or make an herbal nonalcoholic sangria (see page 128).

Fenugreek *(Trigonella foenum-graecum)* is a common herb whose seeds give artificial maple flavor to syrup. It's also used in candies and beverages. It is still in use in Germany as an aphrodisiac drink, made from a decoction of the seeds. This is the only healing herb known to be used as a weapon in war. When Jerusalem was under siege in A.D. 66, the Roman soldiers were ordered to scale the walls of the Jewish city. The common defense in those days to prevent soldiers from scaling walls was to pour boiling water or oil from the top. Jerusalem's defenders, according to Flavius Josephus in *The History of the Jewish War,* added fenugreek seeds to the boiling oil. The seed caused the oil to be considerably more slippery than just plain hot oil.

Ginger *(Zingiber officinale).* Dalziel, a writer in the 18th century, said that in French Guinea and Senegal it was common to chew ginger after chewing a kola nut *(Cola nitida);* the combination was said to be stronger than kola nut alone. Kola nut has a high caffeine content and was historically used for sexual stimulation in African countries.

Ginkgo *(Ginkgo biloba)* is known for treating some kinds of Alzheimer's disease, so says the *Journal of the American Medical Association.* It's been used historically as a memory aid, working by increasing blood flow to the brain. It also increases blood flow to the penis, and more blood means a harder erection. James Duke says that physicians in small studies prescribing between 60 to 240 mg of a standardized ginkgo extract, over a nine-month period, found that 78 percent of the men had significant improvement in erections. He cautioned not to use more than 240 mg because of side effects such as irritability, diarrhea, and overall restlessness.

Mustard *(Brassica* spp.). The seeds of several species of mustard are stimulating. Hot mustard in Asian restaurants will bring perspiration to the forehead, while mustard in stronger form will scorch the skin. The U.S. Army has even used mustard gas as a weapon.

There is little evidence that mustard works as an aphrodisiac, but many medical treatments in earlier centuries were based on irritation as often as healing properties. A man named Davenport in the 1880s wrote that "several cases [of impotence] were cured of atony of the virile member of three or four years' duration, by repeated immersions of that organ in a strong infusion of mustard seed." (Kind of like threatening your penis: "Either you wake up and get to work, or I'm going to torture you in a pot of hot mustard!")

What to Do When You Need a Boost

Other so-called "useful cures" for impotence, taken from the writing of early physicians, include an ointment made of oil and powdered ants' eggs and another of powdered earthworms, which were also mixed with oil and applied to the groin. A more severe treatment was gingerly picking leaves of the stinging nettle plant (wearing gloves, of course), then wrapping the lackadaisical male member in them. Evidently, the theory was that if the member had gone to sleep and wasn't interested in sex, reawakening it by whatever means necessary was an acceptable cure.

My favorite, though, is a remedy from *The Boke* [book] *of Albertus Magnus:* "Perwyunke [periwinkle] when it is beate unto a powder with worms of ye earth wrapped around it and with an erbe called houslyek it induceth love between man and wyfe if it bee used in their meales." So, according to Magnus, you took the periwinkle, some earthworms, and houseleek (hens and chicks), ground up the whole thing, and put it in the food of both the man and woman, and they would become passionate. (It sounds more like a prank played by a fourth-grade boy, doesn't it?)

Richard Allen Miller, in his book *The Magical and Ritual Use of Aphrodisiacs,* lists betel nut, damiana, fo-ti-tieng, ginseng, kava kava, and yohimbe as traditional aphrodisiacs in some countries (with warnings about side effects of many), while Clarence Meyer, in *Herbal Aphrodisiacs from World Sources,* gives a long list of herbs and vegetables that have been used at one time or another for enhancing sexual interest. He says that there is no perfect aphrodisiac, no absolute magic cure, and that diet and a well-rounded life with varied interests and low stress are the best aids to healthy sexual desire.

Nonalcoholic Herbal Sangria

Here's a simple and good-tasting recipe from my book Herbal Cosmetics. *If you and your partner drink this and have love on your mind, who knows, it may get the mood off to a good start, and you can just blame it on the clary sage.*

$\frac{1}{2}$ cup water
2 tablespoons lemon balm leaves, fresh or dry, crushed
1 tablespoon (or 1 small leaf) clary sage leaf, chopped or crushed
1 lemon, thinly sliced
1 tangerine, thinly sliced
2 tablespoons sugar
3 to 4 drops orange extract
1 bottle red grape juice or nonalcoholic sparkling wine
1 can Sprite or 7-Up soda

1. In the microwave, bring $\frac{1}{2}$ cup of water to a boil. Remove from the heat and add the lemon balm and clary sage. Stir, then set aside to steep.
2. Layer the lemon and tangerine slices with the sugar in a medium-size bowl. Add the orange extract and refrigerate for 1 to 2 hours.
3. Pour the red grape juice or sparkling wine over the lemon-tangerine mixture. Strain the lemon balm/clary sage tea and add it to the bowl. Just before serving, fill glasses with ice, pour sangria nearly to the top, and top off the glasses with the soda. If you want it fancy (after all, this is for love), garnish the glasses with a lemon slice and a sprig of lemon balm or mint.

What about Viagra?

Recently, the drug Viagra has put aphrodisiacs and performance-enhancers back in the spotlight. Some men are taking Viagra even if they don't really have impotence problems. There are side effects, and some men have supposedly died after using the stuff. As a sex "bullet," it works pretty well, but the bullet ricochets and knocks out the heart in a very small percentage of men, say some of the drug's detractors. Are there alternatives, possibly herbal, that are safer?

Several things work, although maybe not as quickly as Viagra, but they probably won't put you at risk while having sex, either. I checked one of my favorite books, *The Green Pharmacy,* by James Duke, Ph.D.;

his down-to-earth, personally-tested information is usually right on target. As a researcher for the U.S. Department of Agriculture, he is a respected authority on medicinal herbs. Here are some of the herbs he says are useful for increasing sexual performance (the physical side of performance — if you're a bumbling fool at getting a date, no amount of herbs will help you fix that).

Duke suggests treating impotence-related problems with diet and herbs. The first item on his list is sprouted fava beans (you sprout them yourself). These beans contain L-dopa, a compound that is used to treat Parkinson's disease. Large amounts can cause a painful, continuous erection, called priapism. While that may be your fantasy, you really don't want that. Duke says that 8 to 16 ounces of the beans, sprouted and not eaten all at once, should give even a limp erection a healthy boost. You can use the sprouts on sandwiches or salads. Note, however, that the Vermont Bean Seed Co. warns, "Persons of Mediterranean descent have a genetic trait which may cause an allergic reaction to fava beans."

What Duke claims is the most useful herbal aphrodisiac is yohimbe *(Pausinystalia yohimbe)*. It's from an African tree bark and there are centuries of folklore about its usefulness for men. But Yohimbe also has unwanted side effects, such as anxiety, elevated blood pressure, flushing, hallucinations, and headache. Some pharmaceutical companies have extracted the active compound (yohimbine hydrochloride) and it is marketed under the names Yocon and Yohimex. Duke suggests these are the better way to take this herb. Ask your doctor, as this is available by prescription, and discuss all side effects before you try it.

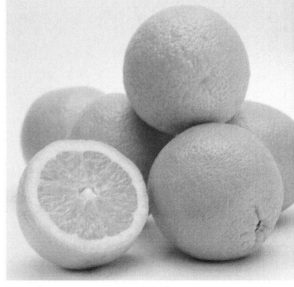

Citrus fruits, such as oranges and tangerines, are not only a healthy snack but also a delicious addition to herbal brews.

Sexual Endurance Tea for Men

Jerry Stamps, in his pharmacy, used to recommend this to men who wanted to maintain their healthy prostate and get a sexual energy boost. It was often just asked for by his customers as "that sex tea you make."

I remember him asking a customer who was buying this, "Do you have high blood pressure?" The customer said he didn't and Mr. Stamps simply said, "It's not recommended if you do, as this can raise blood pressure slightly." He laughingly added, "But of course you want the pressure to rise some during sex."

1 teaspoon damiana
1 teaspoon yohimbe
1 teaspoon licorice (omit if you are on a salt-free or low-salt diet)
1 teaspoon powdered ginseng, root or leaf
1 teaspoon powdered gingerroot
2 teaspoons sarsaparilla
10 drops clove essential oil
10 drops orange essential oil
2 teaspoons cracked or crushed saw palmetto berries

1. Mix all ingredients and store in an airtight container.
2. To use, bring 1 cup of water to a boil. In a cup, pour the water over 2 teaspoons of the herb mixture. Cover with plastic wrap or a lid and let steep for 5 minutes. Drink a cup in the morning and one in the evening. You should start feeling the effects in about 24 hours.

Gently Stiffening Massage Oil

James Duke also recommends essential oils as an aid to erection problems. He suggests a whole-body massage with lotion that contains the essential oils of rose, jasmine, and clary sage. **Note:** *Pure rose essential oil is probably too expensive, even if you can find it. This is the only exception where I use a fragrance oil in place of an essential oil. Jasmine essential oil is also expensive, but do not substitute.*

Here's a mixture I put together based on Duke's suggestion.

2 ounces almond oil
1 ounce apricot oil
4 to 6 drops clary sage essential oil
4 to 6 drops jasmine essential oil
4 to 6 drops rose fragrance oil

Combine the oils in a small container and shake to mix. Warm the oil, the room, the towels, and the massage table. The person giving the massage should shake the oil briefly, then give you a full body massage. The setting, the music in the background, the time spent, the fragrance of the oil, the very good massage — this thoroughly awakens a sleeping member for lots of guys.

The Power of Oils

Dominic Fabis, a massage therapy instructor at the White River School of Massage in Fayetteville, Arkansas, says he prefers to use massage oil without fragrance. "I never got into the aromatherapy thing myself," he said. "My favorite blend of oils is half coconut (not scented like coconut, but the real thing) and half avocado oil. It makes for a very light oil that is full of vitamins that are good for the skin and has no scent. I've used some oil with lavender added and some prepared blends with arnica, but have always come back to rather plain, unscented oils from vegetable, fruit, or nut origin."

Encourage Erotic Dreaming

Another treatment for lack of sexual interest or activity is dream therapy. Dreams can be changed or manipulated by the use of fragrance. The nose and the brain seem to be closely connected. A familiar fragrance can evoke an instant memory before the reasoning part of the mind has a chance to analyze it. Just a whiff of a perfume as you are walking along the street, something you smelled in high school but not since, can instantly evoke the memory of a first date. The smell of roses may remind you of your great-aunt or your grandmother. I've researched, experimented, and played with the ways that fragrance affects memory and dreaming for almost 20 years, resulting in three books on dream blends, and have accumulated scores of dream formulas. Dream therapy is not hocus-pocus but simply based on how the mind perceives and reacts to certain fragrances.

Romance Novel Dream Blend
(As in the Hot Muscle Stud Holding the Buxom Babe on the Book Cover Kind of Dreams)

Here's an erotic formula from my latest book, Making Herbal Dream Pillows *(Storey Books, 1998). If you think you don't dream at night, or think you never have sexual dreams, try this. Some of the ingredients will sound a bit odd, but try the mix. Everything's there for a purpose and I've had excellent results. Unless your nose has quit working, or you are a heavy smoker and have lost much of your sense of smell, this blend is likely to evoke some interesting, colorful, and sensual dreams.*

Note: *All herbs should be dried, cut, and sifted, or cut in small pieces, not ground. The roses and calendula flowers can be whole or just petals. If you are allergic to plants in general or sneeze when using the dream blend, discontinue sleeping with it. Otherwise, it's a healthy blend.*

2 cups roses
4 cups calendula flowers
4 cups rosemary leaves
1 cup lemongrass leaves, cut in short pieces
1 cup sweet woodruff
½ cup mugwort
1 tablespoon spearmint

1 tablespoon marjoram leaves (not ground)
1 teaspoon whole fennel seeds
1 lemon geranium leaf ('Mable Grey' works well, or
   substitute 1 tablespoon lemon verbena leaves)
1 piece of cinnamon bark, about ½ inch long,
   broken up
Small pinch (what will fit on the top of your
   thumbnail) of commercial chili powder

1. Place all ingredients in a zipper-lock bag and mix well. Close the bag and leave for at least two days to let the fragrances blend.

2. Mix again, then take out 3 to 4 tablespoons of the mixture and place it in either a muslin drawstring bag or an old dress sock (clean, of course, without holes). Tie it closed with a rubber band or string and place the little pillow of herbs (this is the dream pillow) in your pillowcase. Don't worry about where it goes in the pillowcase, just tuck it down in the bottom. This isn't potpourri, so the mixture won't have a lot of smell; it's supposed to be *very* subtle. As your head crushes the herbs as you move in your sleep, very small amounts of fragrance will be released.

3. Leave the pillow in your pillowcase for at least 10 days and see if you don't start having some pretty erotic and interesting dreams. And if you are thinking about sex while you dream, it will likely awaken you to the possibilities during the day. I've had some wonderful letters from friends and customers who have tried this mixture and found it lots of fun. And it works on women, too!

Hemorrhoids

Hemorrhoids affect a third of Americans, or about 75 million people, men and women. Basically, hemorrhoids are varicose veins of the anus. Constipation and straining during defecation can bring on a bout of hemorrhoids. The swollen blood vessels can rupture and cause bleeding. The best thing you can do for hemorrhoids, as a man, is to prevent them. Prevent constipation and you've gone a long way toward preventing hemorrhoids.

Prevention as a Weapon

A high-fiber diet that includes fruits and vegetables is the best preventative against hemorrhoids. The Surgeon General urges all Americans to eat five helpings of raw fruits or vegetables a day. Celery, carrots, apples, oranges, bananas, salad greens, and steamed vegetables all fit into that recommendation, and all keep you regular. Follow this guideline and you're pretty much assured that you won't be constipated. (And no, blueberry pie and a can of cherry soda do not count as fruit.)

Another thing you can do to prevent hemorrhoids is to go to the bathroom when you feel the urge instead of putting it off, but don't sit on the toilet any longer than necessary. Don't rush (it's important to relax during defecation; straining from constipation can do damage to the anus's arteries, as well), but don't sit and read three chapters of a book, either.

Herbs That Help Hemorrhoids

The Food and Drug Administration decides what ingredients can go into over-the-counter hemorrhoid medications. Cocoa butter, which is a lubricant, and witch hazel water, which is astringent, are on the official

Help!

How do you know if you are in need of something more than topical help for your hemorrhoids? See your doctor and get his opinion. But what if he says you need an operation to correct the problem? Get a second opinion! There are alternatives to surgery, and in many cases, some very good reasons not to have the surgery.

The tissue around the rectum is sensitive enough to tell whether you are about to pass a solid or a liquid during defecation, and that's information you want to have, and that could be lost with surgery. If your doctor tells you that you need surgery for hemorrhoids, ask about banding the swollen veins. In that procedure, the doctor wraps a miniature rubber band around the hemorrhoid to cut off the blood flow, and it eventually dries up and falls off. Colorectal surgeons are the ones who generally do this procedure, so don't be afraid to ask for a second opinion before you opt for surgery.

list. So are menthol (from peppermint oil), juniper tar (from the juniper tree), and camphor (from the camphor tree, or a synthesized version).

There are other herbs, however, that have a long and accepted use for hemorrhoids. Goldenseal, plantain, chaparral *(Larrea mexicana* and *L. tridentata), comfrey, psyllium *(Plantago ovata),* aloe *(Aloe vera),* and others have all been used topically to treat this painful swelling.

Herbal Sitz Bath

One hemorrhoid treatment, which has some merit for easing the pain, is a sitz bath. A sitz bath can be a whole tub of water you soak yourself in, or a small tub in which you put just your bottom. The trick is to get the affected area, your anus, immersed in an herbal soak for at least 10 minutes.

> 2 cups shavegrass (Equisetum hyemale)
> 1 cup lemongrass (Cymbopogon spp.)
> ¼ cup witch hazel bark (Hamamelis virginiana)
> ¼ cup plantain (Plantago spp.)

1. Mix the herbs and store in an airtight container until ready to use.

2. To use, take out about 1 cup of the mixture and put it in a muslin drawstring bag or tie it in a piece of cloth. Place the bag in a medium saucepan and pour 4 cups of boiling water over the herbs. Let steep, covered, for 20 minutes.

3. Into a washtub big enough to fit your butt, or into a bathtub, pour about 2 gallons of very warm water. Add the sitz bath infusion, squeezing the bag to extract the rest of the liquid. Set the bag aside for another use.

4. Sit down in the very warm water and soak the affected area for 10 minutes. Then apply Hemorrhoid Oil Salve (see page 136). Repeat the bath daily until the swelling subsides.

Hemorrhoid Oil Salve

In The Herbal Handbook, *David Hoffman suggests using a salve made from calendula, chamomile, plantain, St. John's wort, and yarrow after every bowel movement when hemorrhoids flare up. My simplified version is helpful for shrinking swollen tissues.*

You can use cocoa butter instead of the almond oil for a thicker paste, but if you use cocoa butter it should be melted slightly first for a few seconds in the microwave before adding the herbs, then set the mixture aside for 7 to 10 days before using. **Note:** *This can stain underclothes some, but the stains will wash out with detergent and bleach.*

> 1 tablespoon chamomile (Matricaria recutita)
> 1 tablespoon yarrow (Achillea millefolium)
> 1 tablespoon plantain (Plantago major)
> 1 tablespoon St. John's wort (Hypericum perforatum)
> Enough almond oil or warmed cocoa butter to mix

1. Put the herbs into a food processor and blend until powdered (if you can find all of the herbs in powdered or ground form, use those instead). Keep blending until you have a relatively fine dust. Sift or pick out any stems that didn't disintegrate (trust me, you don't want to omit this step).

2. Pour in a small amount of the almond oil or cocoa butter to make a thick paste. Put the mixture into a small container with a lid. This can be used immediately, but will be considerably stronger and more effective if allowed to set for several days.

3. To use, apply to the affected area immediately after the sitz bath, then again every time immediately after defecation.

"Bugs"

There are all kinds of bugs. If they're good bugs, we call then beneficial insects and we expect them to live in the garden. It's when a man finds insects living in the area below the belt that he gets really nervous. A guy's mind might go back to grade school and the "cooties-on-the-toilet-seat" era of childhood. Children deal with fear of the unknown by inventing cooties. Do they really exist and can they really bite you on the butt while you're sitting on the seat? Do they really pole-vault from toilet seat to toilet seat, looking for a crotch to infect?

Getting Rid of Crabs

Crabs are a more specific malady than the generic, fear-inspiring (and nonexistent) cootie of childhood. Crabs, or more precisely crab lice or pubic lice, are small insects that live in pubic hair. While it is remotely possible that you could get them from a toilet seat, the common way of picking up this parasite is from sleeping with someone who has them, or from sleeping in someone else's bed or sleeping bag. You may choose to claim you got them from a toilet seat, but deep down, you and I know they came from someone else's bed.

Crab lice are tiny, pinhead size, and attach themselves to the base of pubic hair; they seldom live anywhere else. The first sign of crabs is itching. You might notice that you're scratching your groin area more than normal, that you wake up at night scratching. If that happens, take a good look in bright light. Examine the spots where the itching is. You can usually see crab lice with the naked eye; they can even be felt with the finger or thumbnail as tiny bumps at the crotch-hair base.

Now that the crabs have your full attention, you're ready to get rid of them at the earliest possible moment, right? More than likely, if you're like most guys, you won't sleep well until you know you *are* rid of them.

I've read accounts in historical books about men on the Santa Fe Trail having crabs so bad that to stop the itching, after trying everything else, they rubbed themselves with gunpowder and set it off. That just demonstrates how intense the itching can become and how near to insanity the sensation can drive a person. I've heard of men using lye soap, kerosene, turpentine, hot pepper, and all kinds of other caustic, painful, and useless methods. Today, however, you simply need to visit your neighborhood pharmacist. There are several over-the-counter

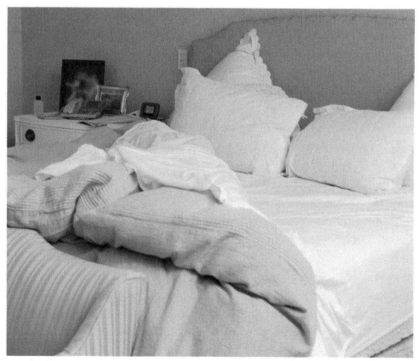

When using a lice treatment, be sure to launder clothes and bedding, too.

preparations that will rid you of your crotch-hitchhikers. Don't be surprised, however, if when you go to the counter to pay for your purchase, the cashier steps back just a little as she hands you the receipt.

Medicine for What Ails You

Supposedly, around 10 million Americans do battle with lice each year, a figure that likely represents head lice and body lice combined (and head lice don't crawl downward to your groin; they're specialized pests that inhabit only their own favorite area). The most common product for controlling the vermin is Kwell. While the skin is still dry, pour some Kwell into your hands, and lather up any affected area — every square inch from your navel down to your upper legs, front and back. Check the directions, as they probably suggest leaving the Kwell on for 2 to 3 minutes before washing it off in the shower. You'll need to repeat the treatment, according to the instructions on the bottle, in a few days. Some people consider Kwell to be toxic, but the results it produces are fast and excellent. Make the choice for yourself.

Then the real work begins. Launder all the bedclothes, even the mattress cover and blankets. A trip through the washer and dryer eliminates the critters (this is better than the process of *boiling* everything for 10 to 20 minutes, which was the recommendation years ago for bedclothes). Any clothing you have worn, or even think you might have worn, since the lice attack must be laundered or dry-cleaned, along with towels, washcloths — anything that might contain more of the little culprits.

Crab lice aren't difficult to get rid of, but you do have to be careful not to put clothes back on that haven't been laundered once you've treated your body for the bugs. Head lice are more difficult to get rid of, and people sometimes shave their head to be sure the eggs are gone. You don't need to shave your groin; simply follow the directions on the bottle of medication and give the area a second treatment to make sure any eggs are killed.

Herbal Alternatives

There are herbal alternatives to Kwell or Rid (another lice medication); however, they require repeat applications over several days. Neem *(Azadirachta indica),* from the neem tree, combined with turmeric *(Curcuma longa),* has shown some potential in the treatment of body lice. You may find organic products in the health-food store that contain these two herbal compounds and might consider asking a clerk for his advice on nontoxic methods of removing body lice. But don't put it off: The longer you wait to get rid of the parasites in your pubes, the more difficult they'll be to eradicate.

Butt Itch

Athletes, construction workers, and campers often get a condition pharmacists used to simply call butt itch. It's brought on by heavy exercise and poor hygiene. A daily bath keeps this from being a problem, but sometimes when bathing isn't regular due to lack of opportunity (as in camping) or from downright laziness, the poor hygiene causes bacteria to grow, and itchy butt develops near the tailbone.

What to Do

When the area has significant bacterial growth, soap and water alone won't clear it up. You can pour some hydrogen peroxide on the area a couple of times a day after bathing and that sometimes will make it go away. I've heard guys say they've poured rubbing alcohol on the problem (now, there's something that lights up your eyes and makes you grateful that no one saw you do such a stupid, and painful, thing). There are a few other solutions. The key is to be consistent in your treatment, or you're simply inviting the infection to come back.

The Blue-Jeans Dilemma

Just one more word about below the belt. Not all men come in the same size. If we did, there would be even more competition for significant others than there already is. But what about a guy with a big butt or no butt at all? How does he ever find a good pair of blue jeans? The Levi's jeans company has a solution. If your butt doesn't fit into an off-the-rack pair of jeans, for about $55 you can have a custom-made pair of Levi's. Call 1-800-872-5384 to find a store near you that will take your measurements, show you fabric samples, and send your made-to-fit jeans on their way.

Buttcrack Ointment

This formula is from my now-deceased pharmacist friend, Jerry Stamps. I checked with my cousin Glenn Foster, a pharmacist in Tennessee, and he updated Jerry's formula for easier use. The ingredients should be available in any drugstore that does compounding (mixing salves, oils, etc.). Here's the combined formula.

Note: *It's important that the Peru balsam and castor oil be blended very well in the beginning to avoid the mixture's separating. It is also important to add the ingredients in the order they are listed.*

> $\frac{1}{2}$ teaspoon Peru balsam
> $\frac{1}{2}$ teaspoon castor oil
> $\frac{1}{2}$ ounce (15 g) boric acid ointment
> 1 ounce (30 g) zinc oxide ointment
> $\frac{1}{2}$ ounce (15 g) aloe vera cream (or substitute
> $\frac{1}{2}$ teaspoon aloe vera gel)
> $\frac{1}{8}$ teaspoon oil of wintergreen

1. In a mixing bowl, blend the Peru balsam and the castor oil, adding just a little bit of each, stirring, then adding a bit more. These have to be mixed thoroughly before proceeding.

2. Mix in the boric acid and zinc oxide. The mixture should have a uniform color with no white showing (or else you need to continue mixing).

3. Mix in the aloe vera cream. Again mix very well, then slowly add the oil of wintergreen, stirring constantly. The process is a bit messy, so do it slowly. The mixture should be stable (that is, not separate) for about 30 days, and can be kept longer if refrigerated.

4. Wash the affected area daily and apply a small amount of Buttcrack Ointment two or three times a day.

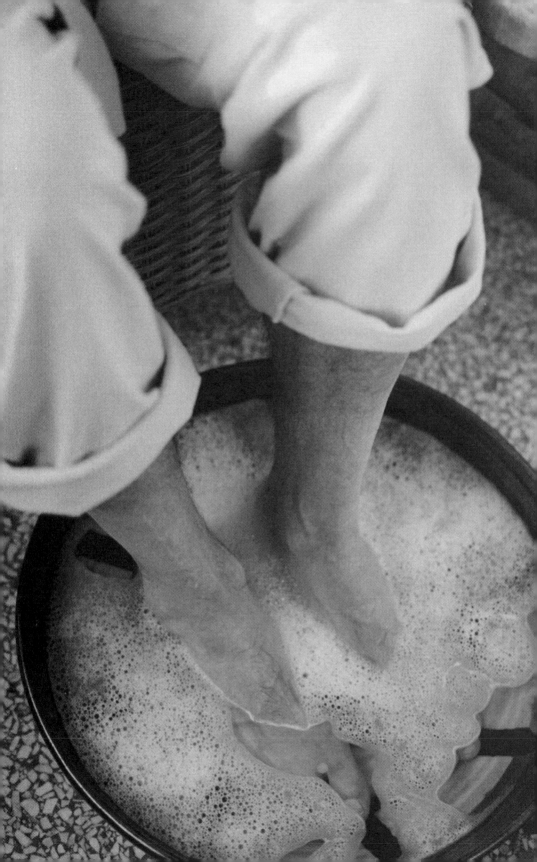

Chapter 5

hands, arms, feet, and legs

■ FLOATING THE BUFFALO RIVER

For many years I organized a float trip for a bunch of guys. It regularly consisted of 15 to 25 friends from as far away as Washington, D.C., Georgia, Texas, elsewhere. We all looked forward to getting together each spring and the float trip was always on the Buffalo National River, which in springtime goes tumbling down the steep mountainsides and roaring through the narrow limestone valleys of the Ozark Mountains. We even had goofy T-shirts made for everyone with our logo of a guy next to an overturned canoe and the words *All Men's Annual Buffalo River Float Trip and Uncomfortable Camp-Out.*

The Buffalo National River was the first in the nation to be designated a National Riverway, and it has been protected and preserved for more than 30 years. It is one of the best white-water rafting rivers in the central part of the United States, surpassed only by the mean and tenacious Mulberry River in spring.

I like the Buffalo River for white-water canoeing because there is enough variety to keep the heart of a novice, as well as that of an experienced canoeist, pumping hard and fast. And the scenery! Imagine 500-foot cliffs with primitive trails along the summits, waterfalls that tumble a hundred feet down cliffs with elegantly twisted, ancient ashe juniper trees that *National Geographic* magazine claims have been dated to more than 950 years of age. Native azaleas and dogwoods, along with hundreds of kinds of wildflowers, mosses, and ferns, turn the oak, hickory, pine, and cedar woods into the most colorful and peaceful spring display that you can imagine.

Our annual men's float trip and camp-out always took place in late March or early April. The water is excellent then, crashing down the canyons and tumbling over the stream's boulders in a rampage of white-water current. The flowers are in bloom and, more important, there aren't many people on the river then.

My favorite float is what we locals call "Ponca to Pruitt" — two approximately 11-mile stretches, putting in at Ponca, Arkansas, camping overnight halfway down, then taking out at the Pruitt access area. Taking two days isn't really necessary, but it isn't speed and quick time that brings us together. It's the challenge, the time to hike and visit and be together as friends, that calls us back each year.

Those of us who have gone rafting on the Buffalo together every year have developed a ritual. Off to the side of the river there is a 2½-mile trail that you can take, leaving the canoes and walking up to Hemmed-in Hollow.

Hemmed-in Hollow is the upper end of a long, deep valley, cut by a small stream flowing downward at sharp angles to join the Buffalo. The trail leads upward, crossing and recrossing the water, winding around ancient moss-covered boulders through the pristine woods. At the summit, a narrow waterfall rushes over a ledge 80 feet high, with enough space beneath the overhang for a campsite if it weren't perpetually wet.

In our annual ritual, everyone strips off everything he is wearing — boots, socks, and hats included — and one by one, with the rest as witnesses, like a crowd of unruly hecklers, walks over the shale pile and into, then under, the not-so-gentle waterfall. Each guy gets cheered on as he stands, letting the pounding weight of the falling water beat his skin like an angry masseur.

I've stood under that waterfall numerous times, covered with goosebumps, chilled to the bone, giddy with the satisfaction that I have performed our rite of spring once again, a baptism in the natural wonder of life. Standing there, with the icy water falling, I feel more alive than I've felt for the entire previous year. Novices will say, "Naw, I don't think I wanna do that," but unwritten law states that the float cannot continue until each man has washed naked in the icy waterfall. It's often those very guys who come back the next year and insist that everyone repeat the waterfall ritual.

One year, my friend David and I decided we would canoe together. David has been canoeing for most of his life. He is good in the canoe, doesn't get rattled easily, and he and I took the rapids well, knowing how each other would react, intuiting how the other would steer and paddle. It's always very satisfying to canoe with someone who knows his stuff, and David and I were having a great time together.

We decided we would bring up the rear of the canoe line. There were about 18 of us in nine canoes, and David said we could help anyone who had turned over. "And besides," he said, "I'd just as soon not hurry. I've been looking forward to this trip all year and I'm anticipating stopping often and hiking along the way."

The river flattens out considerably soon after a set of particularly rough rapids, and you can float along for some distance without much effort other than some light steering with the paddle. Boulders seem to rise out of the water, and many are aluminum-coated on top, attesting to the shallowness of the water in that stretch. The current is surprisingly swift there, even if the water is only about 18 inches deep, and I was keeping the canoe headed into the current with my paddle from the back.

Suddenly a rock that neither of us saw caught the front of the canoe, causing the boat to lurch crosswise of the current. I stepped out of the canoe to push it off the rock and re-angle it with the river. But in a split second the change in weight caused the canoe to flip and fill with water. I stood there for seconds, too stunned to speak, amazed at my predicament. The current had sunk the canoe in the blink of an eye, faster than either of us could comprehend what had happened.

What was worse, the weight of the water-filled canoe had pinned my leg against a duffel-bag-sized rock. A canoe full of water weighs hundreds of pounds; a water-filled canoe catching river current full force probably weighs around a ton, enough to snap a leg in two.

I'm not sure what David did, and I don't think he is, either, but somehow he changed the angle of one end of the canoe by tearing away at a boulder with his hands, and got enough of the water weight off my leg so that I could pull it out.

After dragging myself to the edge, I sat on the bank, feeling my leg. It was so cold it was numb. It was blue. But it wasn't broken! I sat and got my breath back while David maneuvered the canoe so that we could empty out the water and retrieve our gear. I was very grateful, thankful that I could still walk. After a short rest, I was ready to go again.

We'd stowed much of our stuff in 5-gallon plastic buckets with tight lids, tying them together in the canoe. The rest of our gear was in double plastic garbage bags, so nothing was lost, not even my camera equipment. Within minutes we were loaded up and heading downriver again, seriously grateful to be all in one piece. My leg ached like hell, throbbing as the warmth came back. But from that trip I learned a few things about treating sore, strained muscles and bruises.

The Arms and Legs

Let's say you have an office job, sitting at your desk, standing at receptions, using the copier, running for a cab or bus, getting some light exercise only occasionally. Then comes the weekend. You decide to give yourself some outdoor exercise and install the privacy fence you've been wanting in your backyard.

All Saturday morning you dig postholes along the boundary of your back lawn. You mix up some cement and tamp a post in each hole. You're really enjoying the physical work and by Saturday afternoon you're ready for the first frame boards. By evening you're bushed, but you've gotten pretty far along in the project.

Then comes Sunday morning. You can barely move. The shoulder you hurt playing football in high school is acting up big time. Your back aches, the back of your legs are stiff and sore. You moan at the mirror, "Gee, I didn't know I was so outta shape."

Treating Aches and Pains with Herbs

There are several herbs that are beneficial for easing sore muscles, especially when used in a hot pack or, better, in a tub of hot water. Herbs such as marjoram and thyme are antiseptic and warming to muscles, while plantain (*Plantago* spp.) is cooling and helps ease swelling. Herbs for warming the skin, as in arthritis, include mustard seed, cayenne, and nettles (*Urtica* spp.). Arnica (*Arnica* spp.) is very useful on sprains, sore muscles, and bruises, as long as the skin's not broken.

Long Creek's Sore-Muscle Soak

Here's my favorite sore-muscle soak. If you work out or play hard, you might want to make up a batch of this to have handy when you experience soreness or pain (or get your leg pinned under a canoe). The mixture, which will keep a year or more when stored in an airtight container, is the best thing I've ever found for very sore muscles. You can even apply it damp in a drawstring bag, directly on sore muscles, in a tub or not.

A single clean sock makes a good bag for muscle-soaking herbs. We've all got single socks, the mate lost somewhere in the great unknown between the laundry room and the sock drawer. Just put the bath blend in the sock (no holes, of course) and stretch a couple of rubber bands around the twisted top. I've had lots of letters from people who've used this mixture, and I've been making this for customers for a decade.

Note: *All herbs should be dried.*

> 5 cups whole rosemary
> 2 cups chamomile
> 2 cups shavegrass (*Equisetum hyemale* —
>   don't substitute another variety)
> 2 cups thyme
> 2 cups marjoram
> 1 cup calendula
> 1 cup spearmint
> 1 cup catnip
> 1 cup lavender
> 4 cups Epsom salts

1. Combine all ingredients and store in airtight container.
2. When ready to use, take out 1 or 2 cups of the Sore-Muscle Soak and put in a drawstring bag; 4 x 6 inches is a good size. Tie bag closed and place it in a bowl. Start hot water running in a bathtub.
3. While the tub fills up about halfway, pour 2 cups of boiling water over the drawstring bag. Let the hot water soak into the herbs for about 10 minutes, then pour the bag and the water into the tub. Get in and soak the sore body part for at least 15 minutes. A single bag of the blend is good for two or three uses.

Portable Muscle "Soak"

What about body parts that you can't soak, or if you're dealing with something like carpal tunnel syndrome? If you're getting physical therapy, ask your therapist whether he or she has any objections to an herb soak (most will encourage you to use one). When you get the go-ahead, take the herbs to work with you and give yourself some extra muscle-relaxing applications during the day.

Fill the drawstring bag or the sock with 1 to 2 cups of the sore-muscle blend. Dampen the bag and put it in the microwave for a minute or two to make it hot, then apply the bag to whatever area you are treating. Wrap the area in a cloth, towel, or T-shirt and let the herbs and heat relax the area.

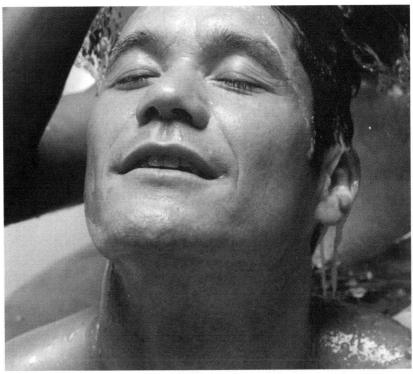

Soaking in a warm herbal bath will help ease even the most uncomfortable muscle aches and pains.

Sore, Tired Muscles Soak

Here's an herb blend that's great as an all-over body soak when you're tired in every joint and muscle. It's even helpful when you've got the flu or just feel lousy. Lock the doors so you won't be disturbed, take the phone off the hook, and make yourself a relaxing warm drink. Then soak yourself in a hot tub with this blend. Soaks have been used by athletes for thousands of years to help rejuvenate their sore, tired bodies.

See Resources for companies that sell muslin drawstring bags. But what if you can't get a bag when you need one? Cut or rip up an old T-shirt into pieces slightly larger than a washcloth. Put the Sore, Tired Muscles Soak into the middle of one of the pieces of cloth. Pull up the corners and sides, and tie it with a piece of string, or use a rubber band. **Note:** *All herbs should be dried.*

1 cup winter savory
1 cup chamomile
1 cup lemon balm
1 cup sweet marjoram
1 cup pine needles, chopped or cut up
  with scissors
1 cup thyme
2 cups rosemary
3 cups Epsom salts
1 cup baking soda

1. In a bowl, mix all ingredients well. Place in a zipper-lock bag or other airtight container.

2. When ready to use, pour 1 to 2 cups of the mix into a muslin drawstring bag. Place the bag in a pan and pour 2 cups of boiling water over the bag. Let it steep while you're filling the tub about halfway with moderately hot (as in "comfortable-but-hot") water. Pour the bag and the liquid into the tub.

3. Soak yourself for 10 to 15 minutes, adding more hot water as necessary. If you're really sore, use two drawstring bags of the mix, filling each with 2 cups of the mix. When finished, squeeze out the liquid and hang up the bags to dry. They can be used a couple more times.

Bath for Bruises and Sore Spots

This bath formula is from my pharmacist friend Jerry. He fixed it for me several times, including after I returned from the canoe trip during which my leg was pinned between the rock and canoe. **Note:** *If life everlasting doesn't grow near you, substitute ¼ cup yarrow* (Achillea millefolium) *and ½ cup sweet marjoram* (Majorana hortensis) *for this ingredient.*

> 1 cup comfrey leaves (see box), cut and sifted
> ½ cup lemon balm *(Melissa officinalis)*
> ½ ounce lobelia *(Lobelia spp.)*
> 1 cup life everlasting *(Anaphalis margaritacea)*
> ½ ounce rosemary leaves *(Rosmarinus officinalis)*

1. Mix together all ingredients and store in an airtight container in a cool, dark place.

2. When ready to use, bring 4 cups of water to a boil and add 1 cup of the bath blend. Simmer on low heat for 5 minutes and strain. Fill the tub with enough hot water to immerse the body part that is sore or bruised. Soak for 20 minutes. Repeat daily until the soreness is relieved.

Comfrey Caution

Comfrey is an ingredient in the above blend. Most current herbal sources recommend not taking comfrey internally and I follow that guideline. Some authorities warn against using comfrey even externally. Personally, I've found this herb to be valuable in healing bruises and injuries, and it's been used throughout herbal history with success. (But if you're curious, look in the library or on the Internet for magazine stories within the last couple of years. Check out information from *Herbalgram* magazine, as well as anything written by Steven Foster, James Duke, and Varro Tyler, all respected authorities on herbs).

Glenn's Scar Lotion

With injuries sometimes come scars. The following formula is from Glenn Foster, my pharmacist cousin in Tennessee. This is good for applying to wounds after they're beginning to heal to keep the scarring to a minimum. It's also helpful for reducing stretch marks after weight loss.

> 2 teaspoons olive oil
> 2 teaspoons wheat germ oil
> 2/3 ounce cocoa butter

1. In a medium saucepan, heat the olive oil and wheat germ oil until well warmed but not hot. Add the cocoa butter and stir until melted.

2. Remove the mixture from the heat and stir until well blended. If you want to make the lotion more salvelike, increase the cocoa butter by 1/3 ounce and follow the same directions. Pour the lotion into a container and allow to cool.

3. Apply lotion directly to wounds that have closed and are beginning to heal. The lotion keeps the area soft and moisturized, cutting down on the amount of scarring.

Hydration Is Key

When doing any kind of exercise, it's important to drink plenty of water. Drink at least 4 ounces of water before exercise, whether it's in the gym or in your backyard, then at least 4 ounces every 20 minutes during the workout, says Felicia Busch, a water-intake adviser for the American Dietetic Association. If you're drinking from a drinking fountain, she says, "an average swallow is about 1 ounce of water; when you're bent over at a fountain, it's a little less, so six swallows comes out about right."

Wake-Up-the-Whole-Body Bath

Maybe you don't want to soak away tired muscles, but want something to tone up your skin. Here's an herbal blend that will make your skin feel really good.

Note: *All herbs should be dried unless otherwise noted. Bulk herbs you buy will likely be "cut and sifted," meaning they are well chopped, but there will be pieces about ⅛ to ¼ inch long. Don't use ground herbs for this recipe; this includes rosemary, which should be used in whole-leaf form.*

Peel of 1 orange
2 cups pine needles (fresh or dry, cut up
    with scissors)
2 cups spearmint
2 cups rosemary
1 cup marjoram (sometimes called sweet marjoram)
1 cup winter savory
1 cup chamomile
1 cup lemon balm
5 bay leaves, broken into several pieces

1. Tear the orange peel into pieces about the size of your thumbnail. Leave it on a plate on the kitchen counter for a few days until it's crisp and dry.

2. In a large mixing bowl, combine the rest of the ingredients with the peel. Store in an airtight container in a cool, dark place. (Just be sure the orange peel and pine are thoroughly dry when you store this; otherwise the blend may grow mold.)

3. Pour 1 to 2 cups of the mix into a muslin drawstring bag. In a saucepan, pour 3 cups of boiling water over the bag, and let it steep while you fill the tub about halfway with moderately hot water. Pour the bag and the steeping liquid into the tub.

4. Soak yourself for at least 10 minutes, adding more hot water as necessary. The fragrances are relaxing and the essential oils in the herb blend's leaves will leave your skin feeling toned and relaxed.

Romantic Bath for Two

Usually we take a bath to get clean, to feel refreshed, or to soothe our tired, aching muscles. But how about a bath you make for someone else? Want to do something special for the person you share your life with? Here's a blend made especially for two, from dried herbs.

Light some scented candles, have a bottle of a favorite beverage and non-breakable glasses on the edge of the tub, and put on some soothing music. This blend, tied in cloth or a drawstring bag and placed in a tub of hot, sudsy water, is a sure way to impress (and likely surprise) your significant other.

6 tablespoons rosemary
6 tablespoons roses
3 tablespoons basil
3 tablespoons thyme
1 tablespoon catnip
1 tablespoon shavegrass
1 tablespoon calendula
4 tablespoons Epsom salts
2 tablespoons Borax (20 Mule Team Borax is found in the laundry detergent section of the supermarket; or substitute 2 tablespoons baking soda)
12 to 15 drops rose fragrance oil
5 drops clove essential oil

1. Mix together all ingredients in a bowl and store in an airtight container, preferably in the bathroom.
2. When ready to use, take out about half the mixture and tie it up in a drawstring bag, being sure to secure it well (an old sock probably isn't the best choice for a bath bag in this instance). Drop it into the tub and run hot bathwater over it while you are getting your partner ready for the tub, assembling the candles and drinks, and starting the music. You'll want the tub a little less than half full.
3. Add a few drops of liquid hand soap or shampoo for suds, get naked, and from there you're on your own.

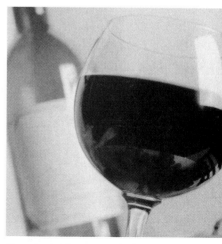

To make a truly romantic bath, drink Nonalcoholic Herbal Sangria (see page 128) as you soak.

Hot-Tub Blend

Here's a body soak for the hot tub for one or more people. It's great for soaking sore muscles and opening the sinuses, as well. The fragrant oils of spearmint and eucalyptus are pleasant, and they mask the smells of the chlorine and chemicals of the hot-tub water. In Japan, where getting in the hot tub with friends and neighbors is common, no one would think of getting into a hot tub without showering first. It's a good practice here, too.

Note: *All ingredients should be dried. From my experience, there seems to be nothing in the mix that would be harmful to the strainers or chemicals of the hot tub (unless you forget to tie the bag closed and let the leaves float around!).*

>   2 cups eucalyptus, whole leaves cut in half
>   or thirds with scissors
>   1 cup shavegrass (Equisetum hyemale)
>   1 cup roses
>   1 cup spearmint or peppermint leaves,
>   whole or cut up
>   ½ cup lavender
>   ½ cup lemon balm

1. Combine all ingredients and store in an airtight container in a cool, dark place.

2. To use, take out 2 cups of the mixture and put it in a drawstring bag, tying it securely to close. Drop the bag into the hot tub about an hour before you get in. That allows the hot water time to soak out the fragrant oils. You can reuse the bag of herbs, or just leave it in the tub for a day or two, then discard.

Hands

Guys do awful things to their hands. Ever watch a car mechanic wash motor parts? Most likely you'll see him with his hands in a pan of gasoline with a scrubbing brush or screwdriver, working at getting the dirt off some greasy metal part. Gasoline is absorbed into his body, and he inhales the fumes, neither of which is healthy. But my point is, we men dunk our hands into all kinds of crappy stuff. Paint, oil, grease, gas, dirt, cement, photocopier ink — you name it and some guy's had his hands in it.

I've had guys come up to me after an herbal program, not wanting to ask their question in an open forum. They'll show me their hands, saying, "Know of anything that will help these?" Generally they have some kind of construction job where they have their hands in mortar mix or wet concrete or chemicals. Their hands are cracked, peeling, red, sore, and obviously painful. Usually they'll say something like, "My wife doesn't even want me to touch her," as if the sore hands don't bother the men at all.

Tips for Healthy Hands

I usually suggest first that they wear gloves, but what they really want is first-aid for their hands. It's perfectly all right — and manly — to wear gloves, use hand lotion, and keep your hands clean and smooth. Use the following formulas to help heal damaged hands.

Treatment for Really Damaged Hands

This treatment sounds pretty strange, even a bit kinky. But it truly is helpful, especially if repeated a couple of times a week. Someone gave me this formula years ago. I found a similar recipe in Natural Hand Care, *by Norma Weinberg (Storey Books, 1998). She says the formula dates back to the Middle Ages, so if it's been around that long, it evidently has been tried many times and found to work. Here's my own version.* **Note:** *You'll need a pair of disposable latex gloves.*

Almond meal is pulverized whole almonds. You can make this in a blender: Just grind the almonds into a fine powder. An even faster method is to combine the dry herbs with the almonds in the blender, the herbs adding bulk and helping the blender motor do the work.

> 1 cup almond meal
> 1 tablespoon comfrey leaf powder
> 1 tablespoon ground thyme
> 1 tablespoon ground parsley leaves
> 2 tablespoons raw honey
> 1 egg
> 1 teaspoon tincture of benzoin (a healing tree resin, available in the pharmacy or health-food store)
> 2 teaspoons vitamin E oil

1. In a bowl, combine the almond with the comfrey, thyme, and parsley, mixing well. Add the remaining ingredients and mix well. It should be a sticky, gooey paste. The mixture is enough for several treatments, so keep the leftovers, covered, in the refrigerator (it will keep only a week or 10 days, so use it up).

2. You may need help with this, and you should apply it right before going to bed. Completely coat both hands with the goo. Have someone hold the gloves open while you put your hands in, covering up the mixture. Leave on the gloves for the entire night.

3. The next day, remove the gloves and discard them. Wash your hands with mild soap and water, dry well, and use a soothing hand lotion to add moisture. Use this mixture two or three times a week until your hands show a marked improvement. Also, use a soothing lotion during the day as often as possible.

Tough Hands Lotion

This is a good hand lotion to use during the day.

> 2 tablespoons castor oil
> 1 tablespoon wheat germ oil
> 2½ teaspoons beeswax shavings
> 1 teaspoon vitamin E oil, 1,000 IU or more
> 10 drops jojoba oil
> ½ teaspoon lecithin
> 15 drops grapefruit seed extract
> 4 drops chamomile essential oil
> 5 drops myrrh-infused essential oil
> 5 drops tea tree oil
> 8 drops lavender oil

1. Combine the castor oil, wheat germ oil, and the beeswax in a microwavable bowl and heat on low until the beeswax is melted.

2. Stir or whisk well, then add the remaining ingredients and mix well again. Continue whisking until the mixture begins to harden to a salvelike consistency. Scrape into a small container and set aside until completely cooled. The mixture should now be heavier than a lotion but a little lighter than a salve.

3. Scoop out a bit of the mixture with your finger and put it in the palm of your hand. Rub your hands all over with this cream, rubbing it in well. This is soothing, and if used on a regular basis, it will soften the skin so that healing can take place.

Smelly Hands

There was an old neighbor fellow, Frank Williams, who fished with me during my summers growing up. He and I kept trotlines in the Osage River and would "run" the lines twice a day. These lines stretched the length of half a block or more, across the river, held down with weights to keep them deep in the water. Every 4 or 5 feet would be a hook, hanging from an 18-inch string, and we would bait all the hooks every day with worms, cut-up fish, crawdads, minnows, whatever we had.

I had a job every summer from the age of 13 on, so if we caught fish in the morning, they would be put into a live box, or strung on a fish stringer in the water. Then when we ran the line in the evening, we would dress the morning and the evening fish at once. Lots of times Frank and I dressed fish all the way up to midnight, getting them ready for my mom to freeze the following day. After dressing fish for hours, our hands would smell like, well, fish.

It's a smell that's not easy to get off, and a smell that isn't easily covered up by another fragrance. I tried dish soap, followed by a vinegar soak, then hand lotion. None of it worked very well, and although my hands were clean, the smell persisted. What can you do about really smelly hands?

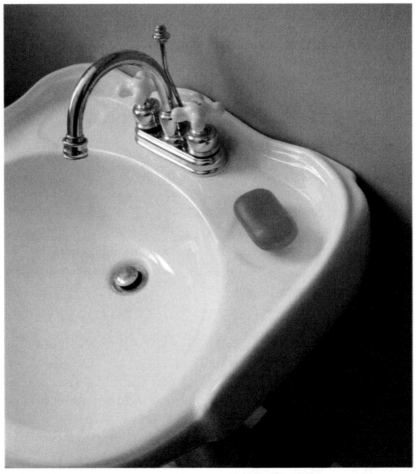

Washing the hands is important, especially if they're dirty or smelly, but excess washing can lead to dryness. Use a moisturizer frequently to combat that "sandpaper" feel.

Fish Odor Remover

Some years back I concocted an herbal mix that does a pretty good job of getting off the fish smell. Bottle some to take along on fishing trips.

Note: *If you make this liquid to take along on a camping trip, add ¼ cup vodka or brandy to the finished product and leave in the lemon pieces. The alcohol keeps the mixture from fermenting or spoiling. Because the alcohol is drying to the hands, you will probably want to use a hand lotion afterward.*

> 2 tablespoons lovage
> 2 tablespoons lemon verbena leaves
> 2 tablespoons spearmint or peppermint leaves
> 1 tablespoon rosemary leaves
> 1 tablespoon sage leaves, or rubbed or ground sage
> 1 tablespoon thyme
> 1 tablespoon lavender flowers
> ¼ fresh lemon, including peel, sliced

1. Mix together everything except the ¼ lemon and store in an airtight container.

2. To use, take out ½ cup of the herb mixture and combine it in a saucepan with 2 cups of boiling water. Simmer the herbs, covered, for 5 minutes.

3. Add the lemon. Let the mixture steep, covered, for another 10 minutes, or even overnight. Strain and discard the herbs. Soak fishy hands in the liquid for 3 minutes. Don't rinse. Dry your hands as usual.

Smoothing Out the Rough Spots

My mom's old standby hand lotion was rose water and glycerine. It felt really great but I wasn't excited by smelling like roses. Hand lotion is very important, however, if you expect that cracked, dried skin to heal. Sure, you could go out and buy one of those chemical-laden products sold at every drugstore or market, but wouldn't you rather use something all-natural and simple to make?

Mom's Expanded Healing Lotion

I've adapted Mom's recipe to be a bit more masculine, but either way, the fragrance evaporates quickly. Glycerine is available in the pharmacy and you can find rose water from the mail-order sources in this book. Rose water soothes and heals besides adding scent — but not the heavy, flowery fragrance that characterizes so many women's lotions.

The lotion adds moisture to hands but doesn't leave a greasy feeling. And the white thyme oil is great for healing small cuts or scratches. This lotion is also nice on feet, arms, knees, and elbows, and even on the face after shaving.

> 1 ounce glycerine
> 1 ounce rose water
> 5 drops spearmint oil
> 5 drops white thyme oil

1. Mix together all ingredients in a bottle. Shake well.

2. To use, shake well and pour out a few drops into your hands. Rub hands together to disperse the lotion, and massage it in.

Pine Needles

You can use dried pine needles (available by mail or from a health-food store) in your formulas; however, fresh ones (or freshly dried) are better by far. If you have access to a pine tree, simply cut a couple of small limbs, about the size of a toothpick, and snip the needles, even some of the wood, with scissors or pruners. The pieces should be about a half-inch long. Dry them briefly, or use them fresh in a bath blend.

Pine is soothing and pleasant on the skin, and is even used in soap. Grandpa's Pine Tar Soap has been around for about a century, and is used to combat skin eruptions and rashes, and just to soothe the skin overall.

Honey and Herbs Lotion

This hand lotion was inspired by Stephen and Deb Pouech of Herbs 'n Honey in Stafford Springs, Connecticut, and found in the book Natural Hand Care, *by Norma Weinberg (Storey Books, 1998). It's soothing and pleasant due to the beeswax. I've adapted their recipe to be less fragrant by eliminating the herbal oils and using fresh rosemary and thyme instead. Because the microwave is faster, I have changed the directions for heating the ingredients.*

The honey is a natural antiseptic and the beeswax smooths and softens your hands. The rosemary and thyme add a nice fragrance and are soothing and healing, as well. It's an excellent lotion for daily use. This makes about 12 ounces of lotion and you can pour it into a plastic squeezable bottle.

> ½ cup sunflower oil
> ½ cup almond oil
> 1 sprig (about 4 inches long) fresh rosemary, broken into smaller pieces (or 1 teaspoon dried herb)
> 1 sprig fresh thyme, any variety, cut up into pieces (or ½ teaspoon dried herb)
> 1 tablespoon beeswax
> ⅓ cup honey

1. Put the oils in a microwavable bowl and heat for about a minute, until hot but not boiling. Remove from the microwave and add the herbs. Cover with plastic wrap and let sit overnight.

2. Remove the herbs, reserving the oil.

3. With a kitchen paring knife or pocketknife, shave the beeswax into small pieces into another microwavable bowl. Cover that with plastic wrap and place in the microwave. With the setting on low (or use the defrost setting), heat until the wax is melted.

4. Warm the oils. When warm, add the honey. Add the liquid to the melted wax and heat briefly again. Don't overheat; you want the wax just melted. Mix well with a spoon or whisk. Set aside to cool so the fragrance of the herbs can permeate the lotion.

5. Pour or squeeze out about ½ teaspoonful of the lotion into your hands and massage in.

Feet

Most guy's feet are hidden nearly all the time, either by boots, sneakers, or whatever. I know guys who say their feet haven't seen daylight in 30 years. Some men wear shoes only when necessary, and I think that may be healthy. It's when your feet are restricted and don't get air that they become hot and sweaty. Bacteria grows easily in shoes and on perpetually moist skin.

Lemongrass Tea

Here's my simple recipe for lemongrass tea, which is a proven fungus-fighter. I prefer to use half a fresh leaf for tea (it's a grass, so a leaf can be about 24–30 inches long; however, this recipe is adjusted for dry lemongrass). The tea is good hot or iced.

1 tablespoon lemongrass
2 cups boiling water
1 teaspoon honey (optional)

In a bowl, pour boiling water over the lemongrass. Cover the bowl and let steep for 5 to 7 minutes. Strain and discard the lemongrass. Sweeten with honey, if desired, and drink over ice or hot.

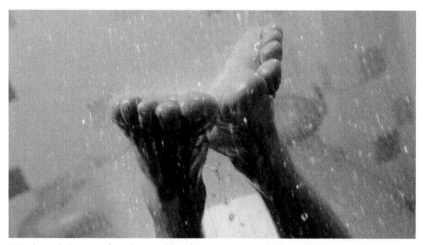

Wash and dry your feet thoroughly after exercise and allow them to get some air. This will prevent the conditions that promote the growth of athlete's foot fungus.

Soak for Athlete's Foot and Nail Fungus

Drinking lemongrass tea helps, but I also like to make a soak for the problem, to speed up the healing. Here's my favorite, which begins to give relief in just a few days.

> 2 cups water
> 2 cups cider vinegar
> ¼ cup lemongrass
> 1 cup shavegrass

1. In two separate pans, bring the water and the vinegar to a boil. As soon as each is boiling, add the lemongrass to the water and the shavegrass to the vinegar. Remove the pans from the heat, and let sit, covered, overnight.

2. Strain out the herbs and discard. Combine the two liquids in a pan large enough for your feet (a plastic under-the-bed shoebox is a good size). Soak the feet twice daily for 10 days, for nail fungus or athlete's feet. Dry off without washing after each soak.

Fighting Athlete's Foot

Here's an easy way to help reduce the risk of spreading athlete's foot fungus to your groin, where it becomes jock itch: After you shower, put on your socks before you pull on your underwear. Even better, cure the athlete's foot fungus and you don't have to worry about socks first.

Dr. James A. Duke, author of *The Green Pharmacy* and a former USDA researcher, recommends lemongrass to fight athlete's foot. He suggests that lemongrass contains natural fungicides that provide healing benefits when drunk as a tea. Applying the steeped, wet leaves directly to the feet is also helpful.

Using Foot Powder

Urban legends are the stuff of long and lively conversations over drinks among strangers in a bar. Someone brings up the story of the stupid lady who decided to dry her poodle in the microwave, then bar patrons line up on either side of the issue and a good debate ensues. Or there's the story of the million-dollar cake or cookie recipe that some lady supposedly stole from Neiman-Marcus, passing it around by mail for decades, and now it's circulating on the Internet.

One of the minor urban legends that I've always liked supposedly comes from the 1960s when everything was counterculture, back-to-the-land, and supposedly chemical-free. It's the story about the sure way to avoid frostbite. As one friend told me at the time, "You just dust a bunch of cayenne pepper into your shoes [socks weren't politically correct back then, except in freezing weather] and the pepper keeps your feet warm."

Great story, really good theory: an all-natural, nonchemical way to keep the tootsies from freezing in frigid weather. The hot pepper just lies there, supposedly warming the feet. I never believed the poodle story and I couldn't quite bring myself to put cayenne pepper in my shoes, or socks, either. Pepper burns skin, whether it's in the eyes or just on an open wound, if moisture is present. (You'll find hot pepper in products like Ben-Gay, Capsaicin, and Icy-Hot, but there it's in a gel or

→ Old-Time Tales

The funny thing about the cayenne pepper story is that it can be found in writings from the Santa Fe Trail period (the 1830s and '40s). Apparently it was a trick played on novice outdoorsmen from "back east." A bunch of guys would be sitting around a campfire in Independence, Missouri, at the beginning of the historic trail, preparing to head to the great Southwest. Veterans would listen to the beliefs and fears (some of them legitimate) of easterner "greenhorns" who were about to embark on their first trip down the trail. Then an old-timer would speak up out of purported kindness and offer the guy a bit of trailworthy advice. "Start out right," he'd say. "Get you some of that there key-enne pepper them wagons bring up from Mexico. Grind it up real fine, then put half a handful in each boot. As you walk out on the trail on cold nights, it'll keep your feet warm. I've used it on every trip!" he'd conclude, the darkness hiding the twinkle in his eyes and the expression on his bullhockey-shoveler's face.

cream base, which brings the warmth without the burning pain of hot pepper against bare flesh.)

But to quote another friend who did try the "remedy": "At first I didn't feel anything different. My feet weren't any warmer, but not any colder, either. But as I walked in the woods, my feet began to sweat and as the moisture was soaked up by the cayenne pepper, my feet began to warm up. Then they began to sting, then they started hurting like hell. I pulled off my boots and socks and soaked my feet in an icy stream. The water didn't remove the sting of the pepper for a while, and I nearly froze my feet in the process. It's undoubtedly one of the stupidest things I've done in years," he said.

Still, I've run across people who swear that they know someone who knows someone who always puts hot pepper in his socks before tramping in the woods. Stephanie Tourles, in *Natural Foot Care* (Storey Books, 1998), mentions it as being useful, and cayenne pepper in the socks may actually work for some people, especially those who have dry feet. But I know for certain that several people have described it to me as feeling like their feet were on fire. Personally, I certainly wouldn't dry my poodle (if I had one) in a microwave, and I won't put cayenne pepper in my socks, either.

Real foot powders, however, are meant to keep the feet dry, and dry feet are more likely to be warm feet. If your feet are sweaty and your

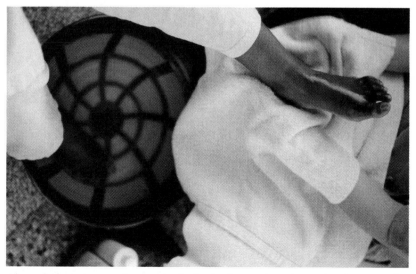

After a foot wash or soak, completely dry the feet and apply an absorbent powder to protect against moisture and odor.

socks get wet, you are more apt to have chilled feet in a short time in winter weather.

Foot powders are made up of a base of absorbent material, often simple cornstarch. Some powders may contain arrowroot, clay, or baking soda, possibly even talc, or a combination of these, but most over-the-counter foot powders are just a cornstarchlike substance, a medicated ingredient, and something for fragrance.

Medicated foot powders, like Gold Bond, contain as their active ingredients menthol (that's mint oil), eucalyptol (eucalyptus oil), and zinc oxide. Zinc oxide is an amorphous powder, ZnO, that's used as a pigment in compounding rubber, an ingredient in making plastics and pharmaceuticals. It has astringent and antiseptic properties that help heal open sores, such as the skin breaks from athlete's foot. It's also used in baby powders to help heal diaper rash. Gold Bond also contains salicylic acid, which is used in the manufacture of aspirin as well as having applications in the treatment of skin problems.

→ The Sandbox

Do you remember that little sandbox thing in the locker room in high school? We never had a name for it beyond "the Box," but everyone had to walk through it at least once a week after showering. It didn't do anything to cure athlete's foot (nor jock itch, even though one big 6'7" bruiser from the football team used to squat and powder his you-know-whats in the dust after each shower; he was big enough that none of us was going to tell him he was wasting his time). What it did do was put some absorbent powder on the feet. Of course walking through it when your feet weren't completely dry was useless. You wound up tracking the stuff across the locker room floor and getting it on your clothes as you pulled them on. I didn't find out what the stuff was for years. Now I know it was basically just cornstarch and baking soda with some talc. Today it's more sophisticated, with active ingredients that actually help prevent athlete's foot and other fungus problems.

Tough Guy's Absorbent Foot Powder

A recipe from The Essential Oils Book, *by Colleen Dodt (Storey Books, 1998), calls for ½ cup arrowroot (or cornstarch, clay, or baking soda) and 8 drops of any essential oil of your choice. That's for a simple, scented foot powder that absorbs moisture. Here's my beefed-up version.*

> 1 cup cornstarch
> 1 cup baking soda (be sure it's baking soda,
>   not baking powder)
> 1 teaspoon zinc oxide powder (if your pharmacy
>   doesn't carry it, ask them to order some)
> 25 drops eucalyptus essential oil
> 20 drops mint essential oil
> 12 drops white thyme essential oil

1. Combine the cornstarch, baking soda, and zinc oxide in a 1-gallon plastic zipper-lock bag. Shake to blend. Add the herb oils by drops to the bag. Zip the bag closed and knead it as you would bread dough, or simply toss it around in your hands for a couple of minutes. Set aside for two days to let the powders absorb the oils. There are two ways to use this.

2. Method #1: Pour the powder into a baby powderlike container (a large plastic salt shaker works well). Stand on a towel and sprinkle some powder on your feet each morning before pulling on your socks.

3. Method #2: Pour the powder into a plastic shoe box (the kind that women store their extra shoes in — it has a lid and is available at a discount store for about $1). Keep the box, lid on, next to the shower. After your feet are completely dry, step lightly into the box, then shake off the excess powder and pull on your socks. It's messy, but it gets more powder on the feet.

Foot Powder for Smelly Feet

You probably know that eating bananas may help control foot odor, but so does washing your socks and feet regularly. But guys whose feet stay damp, or who sweat a lot, can develop seriously foul foot odors that can be difficult to control, regardless of how often they wash their feet. Here's an easy foot powder that you can dust onto your feet in the morning before going to work.

1 cup cornstarch

½ cup baking soda

20 to 25 drops cypress essential oil

(or juniper essential oil)

1. Put all of the ingredients in a food processor and pulse-blend for 10 seconds. If you don't have a food processor, put the ingredients in a zipper-lock bag, close securely, then shake the contents to blend. Store in an airtight container with a shaker lid.

2. To use, dust some on the feet every morning after showering and again in the evening.

Don't Forget to Freshen Up the Shoes

Another way to treat foot odor is to treat the shoes. A salesman from whom I've bought shoes for many years once told me why some kinds of shoes smell worse than others. There are specific standards set by the government regarding the kind of glue used to hold shoes together, "especially sports and jogging shoes," he said. "Those standards don't apply to shoes made in other countries. The glue in those shoes is often made from animal parts, specifically horse and cow hooves.

If you wear sneakers often for exercise or work, chances are they could use a little freshening.

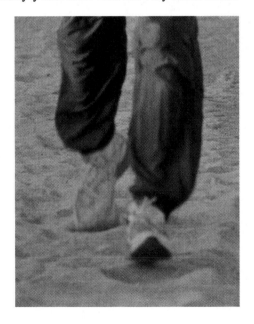

When the shoes absorb moisture over time from workouts and exercise, the glues soften and smells build and make your feet smell. We no longer use those animal-based glues in shoes made in the United States," he said.

Changing shoes helps. Don't wear the same shoes every day. If possible, switch shoes every other day so that they have a chance to dry out, and store your shoes where air can circulate around them (instead of closed up in a box).

Shoe-Stuffers

Some years back I came up with a product that was great for absorbing moisture and odor in any kind of shoes or boots. Over time the discount stores started making a similar product and I ceased offering this to our customers. It's still a really good product and here is my formula. You can make up a batch and keep all of your shoes and boots smelling fresh, as this formula makes enough for several pairs of shoes.

> 2 cups vermiculite (found in the gardening section
> of department stores or in garden stores)
> 2 cups unscented non-clumping kitty litter
> 1 cup charcoal (found in the garden department
> or in any store that sells aquarium supplies)
> 1 cup cedar wood shavings or small cedar chips
> (look in the pet department)
> 1 cup lavender flowers
> 1 cup baking soda
> ½ cup eucalyptus leaves, broken up into small pieces
> ½ cup mint leaves
> ½ cup rosemary leaves

1. Mix together all ingredients in a 1- or 2-gallon zipper-lock bag. Keep in an airtight container until ready to use, as this is highly absorbent and will take up moisture.
2. To use, put about ¾ cup of the mixture into each of two 4 × 6-inch muslin drawstring bags or similar tightly woven bags. Tie closed and place one in each shoe or boot. Keep the bags in the shoes any time you aren't wearing them. The materials absorb any moisture and odor and will last for a year or more, and the pleasant fragrance will be a welcome addition to your closet.

Combating Black Nails: Toenail & Fingernail Fungus

According to *Men's Health* magazine (October 1998), the number of National Basketball Association trainers who have treated toenail fungus is 88 percent. The fungus causes toe- or fingernails to turn black, as if the nail had been hit with a hammer. There are now several kinds of "toxic" (my term) drug treatments on the market to treat this ailment, but if you read the warnings, most can cause severe liver damage if used for more than five to seven days in a row. I've talked with several doctors about the treatments, and most told me that those medicines sometimes work, but just as often don't. And they're expensive — $10 to $20 a pill, with several weeks' worth recommended.

About 15 years ago I started searching for something herbal that was safe and effective to use on skin fungus. I had a fungus, like athlete's foot, only worse, off and on for years. Strangely, though, it affected only my right foot. And my mother had had the same thing, suffering with it for years, also only on one foot. My foot would get dry and flaky, the heel would crack and bleed, and the areas between my toes would also bleed. I'd asked many doctors, including a dermatologist, what it was. Each of them gave me something for athlete's foot and the fungus would go away for a few weeks, only to return again. I decided I wanted a natural and inexpensive cure.

I started looking at *Equisetum hyemale,* greater horsetail (also called scouring rush and shavegrass). Back in the '60s it was claimed to be an organic remedy for fungus disease on roses. I read up on the plant and found that one variety, the one with little fringelike fingers at the joints *(E. arvense),* can cause skin irritation, but that *E. hyemale* had no such warning. Once used as a folk remedy for so-called kidney complaints, it had fallen into disuse. (Consult the *Peterson Field Guide to Medicinal Plants* for an illustration and specific identification, or buy the herb from a reputable supplier.)

I knew that fungus diseases often respond to a change in the pH level of the skin, so I boiled cider vinegar with shavegrass and allowed the mixture to steep overnight. I strained the liquid and soaked my foot 2 minutes daily for 10 days.

To my surprise, the skin problem started clearing up in just a few days. By the end of 10 days, new skin was growing back and the pain and irritation were completely gone.

The next time I used this was on my father, who didn't have an herbal inclination of any kind. In his 80s, he developed black spots on two of his fingernails, which looked like he might have hit the nails with a hammer. One evening, he asked if I had anything herbal for his fingernails. His physician had told him that if the fungus continued, he would have to remove the nails, as there wasn't much of anything else to do (I've since had many people tell me they have had their blackened finger- or toenails removed by their doctor).

I mixed up some of my vinegar-shavegrass solution and told him to soak his fingertips in a shot-glassful every night for 5 minutes while he watched the evening news. In less than two weeks his doctor called to ask me what I had used on my father's fingernails. "I've never seen this fungus clear up so fast," he said. And it didn't return.

Nail Fungus Soak

Since those original formulas, I've had hundreds of people tell me how effective this simple treatment is. For years I've made this up in a kit form, including the recipe and herb, and it's been one of our top-selling products. Here's my recipe.

> 4 cups cider vinegar
> 1 cup shavegrass, dried, cut into pieces

1. Bring the vinegar to a boil and add the shavegrass. Let it boil for about 1 minute. Remove from heat and let sit, covered, overnight.

2. Strain out the herb and discard. Pour the liquid into a plastic shoe box with a lid if using it for feet, or into a small jar or container if using it for hands.

3. To treat toenails, keep a container of the mixture next to the shower. After you have finished showering, step into the plastic box and soak a foot for 30 seconds to a minute. Lightly dry and repeat with the other foot.

4. To treat fingernails, soak all the nails in the solution for 1 to 2 minutes. Lightly dry. Repeat, for feet or hands, daily for 10 days; twice a day is even better.

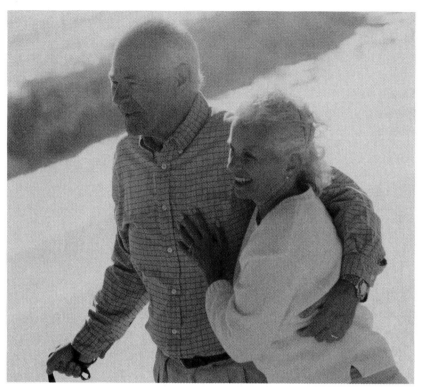

Using herbs in combination with a good diet and an active lifestyle will ensure good health for years to come.

Natural Fungus Killers

Another source, the *Therapeutic Herb Manual*, by Ed Smith of the Herb Pharm in Williams, Oregon, recommends a combination of usnea lichen *(Usnea barbata)*, spilanthes *(Spilanthes oleracea)*, oregano (*Origanum* spp.), Pau d'Arco *(Tabeuia impetiginosa)*, and tea tree oil *(Melaleuca alternifolia)* for other kinds of nail fungus. The Herb Pharm offers this in concentrated tincture form, and recommends it for different kinds of toenail and fingernail fungus, ringworm, and athlete's foot. On the kind of toenail fungus that causes the nails to turn yellow and thicken, a combination of using Herb Pharm's spilanthes-usnea tincture once daily and my shavegrass-vinegar solution is effective for many men.

glossary

The plant materials mentioned here can be purchased fresh from garden centers or dried from some health-food stores and bulk-herb suppliers.

Almond *(Prunus dulcis).* Ground almonds (called almond meal) are used as an abrasive in face and body scrubs to remove dead skin and dirt in pores. Buy whole almonds in the grocery or health-food store, then pulverize some.

Almond oil, sweet. This is a light lubricating oil for the skin, used in good-quality massage oils and hemorrhoid medications. It is an emollient and emulsifier found in creams for chapped hands, lotions, nighttime skin-care products, suntan gels, and makeup bases.

Aloe *(Aloe vera).* The gel that's inside the leaf of the aloe vera plant is one of the best minor burn treatments available. It has antibacterial action, making it useful in healing cuts and small wounds as well as soothing sunburn. You can buy aloe vera gel in the pharmacy or discount store, just be sure you don't get the *juice*.

Alum. Aluminum potassium sulfate is a topical astringent. It helps to stop bleeding, and thus is an ingredient in styptic pencils. Available in pharmacies that carry over-the-counter materials. For an herbal alternative, see yarrow.

Apricot oil. This is a light, fine oil pressed from the kernels of apricots. It is used on sensitive and damaged skin. Apricot oil is rich in vitamins A and B.

Arnica *(Arnica montana).* Arnica is useful in reducing inflammation and external signs of bruising. However, it isn't recommended for broken skin.

Baking soda. Sodium bicarbonate is used in baking, and is good for easing gas pains, as a moisture-absorbing agent, and as a simple tooth powder. Don't use baking powder instead of baking soda in your formulas — they are not the same thing. Baking soda is alkaline, soothing to minor skin irritations.

Basil *(Ocimum basilicum).* An aromatic herb commonly used in Italian seasoning blends, basil contains many antiviral compounds, as well as varying amounts of vitamins A and C. The plant is useful for removing warts, treating bad breath, and easing headaches.

Beeswax. Pure beeswax is used in salve and lotion formulas to make a stiffer, more solid substance. Available in crafts stores in the candle-making section as well as from mail-order sources, but be sure it is food-grade quality.

Borax. Anhydrous sodium borate, borax adds water-softening properties to bath blends that help the soap suds up more. Ask for borax in the pharmacy, or use the 20 Mule Team brand laundry additive, found in the grocery store.

Boric acid. A crystalline compound used as an antiseptic and in cosmetics. Available in the pharmacy as a powder.

Calendula *(Calendula officinalis)*. Calendula is somewhat antiseptic and is used for dry or damaged skin irritations, and bee and other insect stings.

Castor oil. A clear oil extracted from the castor bean plant, *Ricinus communis*. This is a heavy oil and helps to seal in moisture in skin preparations. You can find castor oil in most drugstores.

Catnip *(Nepeta cataria)*. Catnip is a mild tranquilizer; it contains nepetalactone isomers, chemicals that are similar to the constituents of valerian, another sedative herb.

Cayenne pepper *(Capsicum annuum)*. This is a moderately hot pepper that contains capsaicin, a powerful local stimulant that acts to increase blood flow and oxygen to body cells. It produces a feeling of warmth, and is the warming ingredient in many over-the-counter salves, rheumatism rubs, and sports creams.

Chamomile *(Matricaria recutita)*. The plant's oils have been found to work as an antibacterial and anti-inflammatory. And a cup of tea before bedtime helps you relax and fall asleep quicker. Chamomile is also useful as face lotion for soothing oily skin.

Cider vinegar. A dilute solution of acetic acid, obtained from the fermentation of fruit or other vegetable matter. It contains potassium and trace minerals and is used as a preservative, antibacterial, antiseptic, and skin cleanser. Health-food stores are the best places to look for pure cider vinegar, and Heinz makes one that's sold in grocery stores.

Citrus. Citrus fruits, including orange, lemon, tangerine, and grapefruit, are strong astringents, useful in aftershaves and face lotions to combat oily skin.

Comfrey *(Symphytum officinale)*. For centuries this herb has been used to speed healing of wounds on the skin. I find comfrey poultices excellent for skin injuries and in the bath, but it shouldn't be used internally.

Cornsilk *(Zea mays)*. The silk, or "hairs," from an ear of corn are diuretic and used to treat kidney disease and cystitis. Cornsilk is also used in medicine, cosmetics (such as in face powder), and foods.

Cornstarch. A purified starch flour made from corn. Often used as a drying agent to remove skin moisture, cornstarch is found in the grocery store.

Couch grass *(Agropyron repens)*. This herb is used to treat urinary-tract infection, water retention, bladder problems, and kidney stones.

Cucumber. This fruit is an astringent, used for drawing moisture and oils from the skin. It also reduces eye puffiness after a night out on the town.

Damiana *(Turnera diffusa)*. Damiana is used as a flavoring agent in alcoholic and nonalcoholic drinks, frozen dairy products, puddings, baked goods, and aphrodisiac teas and beverages.

Dandelion root *(Taraxacum officinale)*. Dandelion, a strong diuretic, can help ease problems of the bladder and kidney. The latex, or white juice, from a fresh dandelion stem is claimed by some herbalists to be a fairly good cure for warts. Don't use dandelions that have been sprayed with pesticides.

Decoction. A strong tea made by simmering an herb or herbs in water.

Echinacea *(Echinacea* spp.). The herb has been found to help avoid or minimize colds and flu because it boosts the immune system. It is also reportedly beneficial for treating yeast infections and athlete's foot.

Elderberry *(Sambucus canadensis)*. This common roadside plant is useful for cuts, sores, rashes, and insect bites.

Epsom salts. Magnesium sulfate heptahydrate; called simply "salts" in many old formula books. It's an old standby for soaking sore muscles, used by many coaches. Epsom salts is available in pharmacies and most grocery stores.

Essential oils. Essential oil is the extracted oil of a specific plant, and it contains the healing or beneficial constituents of the given plant, in very concentrated form. Don't substitute with fragrance oil, unless specified.

Eucalyptus *(Eucalyptus* spp.). A very aromatic herb, eucalyptus warms the skin and soothes muscles, thus the oil's inclusion in sore-muscle preparations. We use it in hot-tub blends because of the great fragrance. It's also one of the oils in chest rubs, and aids in opening up sinuses when you have a cold.

Fuller's earth. A highly absorbent clay used in powders and absorbent cosmetics. You can order this from bulk-herb suppliers, or find it in some drugstores.

Ginger *(Zingiber officinale)*. Ginger is useful in treating a wide range of problems, including motion sickness, dizziness, nausea, seasickness, dandruff, erection problems, body odor, colds, coughs, and upset stomach. Fresh gingerroot can be found in the grocery store.

Ginkgo *(Ginkgo biloba)*. This herb has received a lot of good publicity for improving memory and treating some early forms of Alzheimer's disease. Ginkgo causes increased oxygen flow to the brain and other parts of the body.

Ginseng *(Panax quinquefolium)*. American ginseng is an adaptogen, meaning that it helps return the body to normal. Research points to its use to increase mental efficiency and physical performance and in reducing the effects of stress.

Glycerin or glycerol. Glycerin is a colorless, syrupy by-product of soap manufacturing, made from the fats and oils of animal or vegetable materials. It is an ingredient in many cosmetics, inks, and lubricants. Vegetable glycerin is available from the pharmacy and is found in many grocery stores.

Goldenseal *(Hydrastis canadensis)*. Traditionally used in tea or as a tincture to treat inflamed mucous membranes in the mouth, throat, and stomach, goldenseal contains berberine, which is antibacterial.

Gravelroot *(Eupatorium purpureum)*. Gravelroot has been used in folk medicine to treat kidney stones, gout, and impotence.

Honey. Honey is an emollient, an antiseptic, and a bacteriostatic. Try to find raw, unprocessed, nonpasteurized honey from health-food stores, for use in salves and lotions.

Hyssop *(Hyssopus officinalis)*. The herb is currently used as a treatment for coughs, hoarseness, and sore throat, and for loosening phlegm; this plant also has a centuries-long reputation as an important wound herb on the battlefield.

Infusion. A tea, made by steeping but not boiling.

Lavender *(Lavendula officinalis)*. A relaxing, fragrant perennial plant that is useful in bath blends and sleep pillows for easing headaches.

Lecithin. Produced commercially from soy beans, corn, or egg yolks, this emulsifier is used in cosmetics, foods, and pharmaceuticals. Available in health-food stores and some pharmacies.

Lemon balm *(Melissa officinalis)*. A mildly lemon-scented herb used in tea, aftershaves, lotions, and soaks for bruises and sore areas.

Lemon verbena *(Aloysia triphylla)*. The leaves of the plant, which can be used fresh or dried, are great for tea, give flavor for a really mean cheesecake, and are a component in aftershave preparations.

Lemongrass (*Cymbopogon* spp.). Lemongrass oil is very effective in fighting several kinds of skin fungus, including athlete's foot. The herb is good in bath blends, helping soothe and heal the skin, as well as in aftershave mixtures. Lemongrass leaves make a pleasant tea.

Licorice *(Glycyrrhiza glabra).* Used in the treatment of a number of problems such as ulcers, smoking cessation, colds, and flu, and included in prostate-reducing teas and tinctures. Avoid if taking high blood pressure medicine or following a salt-free diet.

Life everlasting *(Anaphalis margaritacea* and *Gnaphalium obtusifolium).* This medicinal herb is used in the treatment of wounds and bruises.

Linden flowers (*Tillia* spp.). These flowers are softening and soothing to the skin and used in bath blends and skin soaks. They are also effective as a diaphoretic (producing perspiration), as a tea, and in dream blends.

Lobelia (*Lobelia* spp.). *Lobelia inflata, L. siphilitica,* and *L. cardinalis* are used in bath formulas for soreness. *L. inflata* (and related species) shouldn't be taken internally; the plant has some mind-altering effects that can cause coma and death in some cases. You can buy lobelia through mail-order sources or in your local herb shop.

Lovage *(Levisticum officinale).* A commonly cultivated garden plant in the United States and Europe. Medicinally it has a reputation for increasing urination and expelling gas (a good burp, not the other direction).

Marjoram *(Origanum majorana).* Although it is known mostly as a culinary plant, marjoram's fragrance in dream blends is relaxing, and in bath blends it is soothing and relaxing for the skin. It can speed up the healing of bruises and skin injuries, and is also an ingredient in hair rinses.

Marsh mallow *(Althea officinalis).* The root has been used in folk medicine to treat bladder infections, skin problems, sore throat, and other related complaints.

Mint *(Mentha* spp.). Spearmint or peppermint can be used, as well as most any other pleasant-scented mint. Mint will refresh, cool, and invigorate the skin, and is a digestive aid.

Myrrh *(Commiphora myrrha).* Made into a tincture, myrrh is commonly used to make a mouthwash and gargle for sore throat. It's astringent, antifungal, antibacterial, and antiviral, with cooling and antiseptic properties, making it useful in hand lotions and on wounds and abscesses.

Oatstraw *(Avena sativa).* This herb is known for enhancing stamina. Oatstraw actually is the straw, or stem, of the oat plant.

Parsley *(Petroselinum sativum)*. Parsley is useful in treating bad breath, bladder infections, kidney stones, and, topically, bruises. Parsley has a short shelf life, so replace yours if it's more than six months old.

Pine *(Pinus* spp.). Grandpa's Pine Tar Soap has been used for skin ailments and oily skin and eruptions for a century, and is still available today. The fresh or dried needles and small twigs are relaxing and soothing in the bath blend.

Plantain *(Plantago major* or *P. lanceolata)*. A healing herb useful on wounds, scratches, rashes, and insect bites. It's confirmed (by research) to be an antimicrobial that stimulates the healing process. Traders on the Santa Fe Trail stuffed the green, bruised plant's leaves up you-know-where to treat hemorrhoids.

Raspberry *(Rubus idaeus)*. The leaves are astringent and have been used in treating diarrhea, painful menstrual cramps, and childbirth problems, and for reducing swelling in the body.

Rosemary *(Rosmarinus officinalis)*. Most widely known as a valuable cooking herb, rosemary tea makes an excellent hair rinse for dark hair, and it is a terrific ingredient in herbal aftershaves. Additionally, it is antispasmodic and helpful in treating painful joints and stiff muscles.

Rose water. A combination of distilled water and essential rose oil, used as a flavoring in desserts and as a fragrance in lotions and cosmetics. Be sure when you purchase rose water that it is certified "food grade"; otherwise, it is not to be ingested. Look for it in a health-food store or see Resources.

St. John's wort *(Hypericum perforatum)*. Used as a folk remedy for bladder ailments; topically in oil or decoction on sores, cuts and wounds, and hemorrhoids. Shown to be a sedative and antidepressant.

Sage *(Salvia officinalis)*. Herbalists sometimes recommend sage tea for excessive sweating and to relieve gas pains. It's also used as a throat gargle, as a lotion for minor skin wounds, and in hair rinses and aftershaves.

Salt. Occasionally used as an abrasive in face scrubs; plain sea salt crushed in the blender, rather than table salt, is best for this purpose.

Saw palmetto *(Serenoa repens)*. Known for its ability to shrink enlarged prostate glands, saw palmetto is usually taken as a capsule or tincture for prostate treatment, unless you make a tea. The seed, or whole berry, is also used in tea or a tincture.

Scented geranium *(Pelargonium* spp.). Scented geraniums come in all fragrances, including rose, coconut, cinnamon, citrus, and apple, and are used in potpourris and sachets. Lemon, especially the variety 'Mable Gray,' is good in small amounts in dream blends and for scenting aftershave and body dust.

Shavegrass *(Equisetum hyemale)*. I've found this plant useful in treating athlete's foot fungus and the fungus that causes toenails or fingernails to turn black (see formula, page 171).

Stinging nettle *(Urtica dioica)*. Considered a weed in many parts of the United States, the herb is very useful as a cooked green and in hair preparations.

Stoneroot *(Collinsonia canadensis)*. Stoneroot is used as a diuretic in kidney and bladder ailments, as well as topically for burns, bruises, sprains, and wounds. Do not use the *fresh* leaves internally.

Sweet woodruff *(Galium odoratum)*. In dream blends, this herb adds a feeling of lightness and sometimes flying to the dream. Use the plant in dried form, rather than fresh.

Tea tree *(Melaleuca* spp.). The oil is antiseptic and contains terpenes, which can penetrate the top layers of skin and carry their disinfectants deeper than most emollients. Used to help control dandruff, it is also a component of healing hand lotions. Also useful in treating athlete's feet; just don't take it internally.

Thyme *(Thymus* spp.). Scientific tests have proved thyme's effectiveness as an antispasmodic and cough reliever. Thyme is especially useful for healing cuts or wounds in the mouth. I often drink a strong thyme tea for a sore throat gargle.

Tincture. An alcohol extraction of an herb. The tincture is a concentrated product from the herb and is generally used by the drop or dropperful.

Tincture of benzoin. Benzoin is a tree resin *(Styrax benzoin)* that is an antiseptic and astringent, used to heal inflamed or cracked skin. It helps improve skin elasticity and is also employed as a cosmetic fixative, especially with oils and vegetable fats in formulas. Available in some pharmacies and health-food stores or by mail.

Valerian *(Valeriana officinalis)*. This moderately common garden herb is a natural relaxant with sedative effects. In capsule form, it is helpful before bedtime to relax muscles and encourage sleep. It's also a mild pain reliever and useful for back pain.

Wheat germ oil. Oil extracted from the vitamin-rich embryo of the wheat kernel. Because of the oil's healing benefits, it is often used in lotions and salves. You can find wheat germ oil in pharmacies and health-food stores.

White thyme oil. Essential oil from the white thyme plant *(Thymus vulgaris)*, it's considered healing and helpful for first aid on scratches and wounds. Thyme in the bathwater helps soothe the itch of insect bites. White thyme oil can be bought from mail-order sources and in some health-food stores.

Winter savory *(Satureja montana)* is a soothing and fragrant bath herb.

Witch hazel *(Hamamelis virginiana)*. Available from pharmacies and grocery stores, witch hazel has been used for centuries as a skin freshener and aftershave. Used commercially in pharmaceutical formulas to treat minor pain, itching, and hemorrhoids and to keep muscles limber.

Yarrow *(Achillea millefolium)*. Yarrow is astringent, hemostatic, and anti-inflammatory. A few people have reported mild dermatitis, so try it on a small patch of skin before applying it to a larger area. Yarrow tea makes a pleasant aftershave and closes up the pores quickly. I have often used the yellow-flowered yarrow *(A. filipendulina)* to stop the bleeding of minor cuts.

Yohimbe *(Pausinystalia yohimbe)*. An African folk aphrodisiac known to stimulate erections. There are several side effects (including anxiety, elevated blood pressure, increased heart rate, and headache) from taking the dried bark alone on a regular basis. Yohimbine, the extract of yohimbe, is available by prescription from a physician.

Zinc oxide powder. ZnO is an amorphous white or yellowish powder used in the manufacture of pharmaceuticals and cosmetics. Said by some to toughen or strengthen the skin, and useful in athlete's foot healing powders. Find it in your local pharmacy.

resources

Hand and Body Lotions and Herbal Products

Camden-Grey Essential Oils
8567 Coral Way, #178
Miami, FL 33155
(877) 232-7662
Fax (305) 229-7164
Web site: www.essentialoil.net
E-mail: aroma@bellsouth.net

*An excellent source of massage and
essential oils.*

E. Elan Co.
PO Box 105
Collins, MO 64738
(417) 754-2798
Web site: www.elancompany.com

*Handmade goat's milk soaps, shave
cream soaps, Simply Splendid Hand &
Body Lotion. Catalog $1.*

Evening Shade Farm
Gayl Bausman
RR 2
Osceola, MO 64776

*Handmade goat's milk soaps, marbled
herb soaps, Liberty-Rose Body Lotion.
Catalog $1*

The Herb Pharm
PO Box 116
Williams, OR 97544
(800) 348-4372
E-mail: HerbPharm@aol.com

Tinctures, therapeutic herb manual.

Summer's Past Herb Farm
15602 Old Highway 80
El Cajon, CA 92021
Vegetable-based herbal soaps.

Bulk Herbs

Greenfield Herb Garden
PO Box 9
Shipshewana, IN 46565
(800) 831-0504

*Plants, seeds, supplies, bulk herbs; cata-
log on request.*

Heritage Products
Box 444
Virginia Beach, VA 23458
Food grade rose and lavender water.

Long Creek Herbs (Jim Long's company)
Route 4, Box 730
Oak Grove, AR 72660
(417) 779-5450
www.longcreekherbs.com

*Bulk herbs, dream blends, muslin draw-
string bags, rose water, assorted essential oils, bath blends, sore-muscle soaks,
frankincense, myrrh, and related supplies. Catalog $2, refundable with order.*

Nichols Garden Nursery
1190 North Pacific Highway
Albany, OR 97321
www.pacificharbor.com/nichols/
Bulk herbs, herb and vegetable seed and plants, beer-making supplies. Catalog on request.

Our Family's Herbs & Such
702 Llano
Pasadena, TX 77504
(800) 441-1230
Bulk herbs and supplies. Catalog $1.

Richters Herbs
Goodwood, Ontario
LOC 1A0
(905) 640-6677
www.richters.com
Educational catalog of plants and bulk herbs. Catalog upon request.

Rosemary House
120 South Market
Mechanicsburg, PA 17055
(717) 697-5111
Bulk herbs, plants, books. Catalog $2.

Teeter Creek Herbs
Bob Liebert
Route 5
Ava, MO 65608
High-quality tinctures and herb extracts. Catalog upon request.

Vermont Witch Hazel Company
4415 Ponca Avenue
Toluca Lake, CA 91602
(818) 766-4046
www.mallsurfer.com/shop
and
113 Main
Windsor, VT 05089
(802) 674-5060

Educational Resources

American Association of Kidney Patients
(800) 749-2257
Open weekdays, 8:30 A.M. to 5:00 P.M.

American Diabetes Association
Web site: www.diabetes.org

American Society of Plastic and Reconstructive Surgeons
(800) 635-0635
Web site: www.plasticsurgery.org

Curing Heartburn HotLine
American College of Gastroenterology
(800) 478-2876

Foundations in Herbal Medicine
Tieraona Lowdog, M.D.
112 Hermoa, SE
Albuquerque, NM 87100

Gastrointestinal Problems Hotline
(888) 964-2001

International Foundation for Functional Gastro-Intestinal Disorders (IFFGD)
(888) 964-2001
Web site: www.iffgd.org.

Johns Hopkins Health Information
Web site: www.intelihealth.com

Northeast School of Botanical Medicine
PO Box 6626
Ithaca, NY 14851

The director of this school is 7Song, a practicing Western Clinical Herbalist who specializes in men's health and herbal first aid. 7Song has taught at the California School of Herbal Medicine and the Southwest School of Botanical Medicine, and is a frequent speaker at conferences throughout the United States. He offers herbal programs and classes designed to give in-depth, hands-on, comprehensive understanding of herbal medicine.

People's Pharmacy
Web site: www.peoplespharmacy.org

SportsDoc
Web site: www.medfacts.com
/sprtsdoc.htm

Consumer Affairs Office
T. N. Dickinson Co.
PO Box 319
East Hampton, CT 06424
(860) 267-2279

Supplier of good quality witch hazel.

The Duct Tape Page
Web site: http://204.255.212.10
/~jthorsse/duct.html
e-mail: jthorsse@bcpl.net

Kirk's Coco Castile Soap
(800) 825-4757
or look in better grocery stores

Levi's
(800) 872-5384

Sunglass Hut
(800)-SUNGLAS
Web site: www.sunglasshut.com

Miscellaneous Sources

Bruce Thorpe
Studio B Pottery
RR 1, Box 1050
Reeds Spring, MO 65737
(417) 272-8775

Maker of the Man's Tea Steeper Mug, $29.95 including postage.

index

other storey books you will enjoy

Herbal Antibiotics, by Stephen Harrod Buhner. This book presents all the current information about antibiotic-resistant microbes and the herbs that are most effective in fighting them. Readers will also find detailed, step-by-step instructions for making and using herbal infusions, tinctures, teas, and salves to treat various types of infections. 128 pages. Paperback. ISBN 1-58017-148-6.

The Herbal Body Book, by Stephanie Tourles. Learn how to transform common herbs, fruits, and grains into safe, economical, and natural personal care items. Contains over 100 recipes to make facial scrubs, hair rinses, shampoos, soaps, cleansing lotions, moisturizers, lip balms, toothpaste, powders, insect repellents, and more. 128 pages. Paperback. ISBN 0-88266-880-3.

Keeping Fitness Simple, by Porter Shimer. This retitled, redesigned edition of *Too Busy to Exercise* offers fun, easy fitness tips that don't involve expensive health clubs or exhausting workouts. 176 pages. Paperback. ISBN 1-58017-034-X.

Keeping Life Simple, by Karen Levine. This easy-to-read book helps readers assess what's really satisfying and then offers hundreds of tips for creating a lifestyle that is more rewarding. 160 pages. Paperback. ISBN 0-88266-94305.

Making Herbal Dream Pillows, by Jim Long. Learn to stimulate emotions and long-lost memories and produce vivid dreams that are exciting, relaxing, or creative. This lavishly illustrated book offers step-by-step instructions for creating 15 herbal dream blends and pillows for custom-made dreams. Also included are the history of dream pillows and their ties to folk medicine and herbal mythology. 84 pages. Hardcover. ISBN 1-58017-075-5.

Natural First Aid, by Brigitte Mars. This book offers natural first-aid suggestions for everything from ant bites to wounds. Readers will also find recipes for simple home remedies using herbs, vitamins, essential oils, and foods. An herb-by-herb section describes the healing properties of common herbs. 128 pages. Paperback. ISBN 1-58017-147-8.

Rosemary Gladstar's Herbal Remedies for Men's Health, by Rosemary Gladstar. Natural solutions to health problems common to men such as low energy, infertility, prostate problems, heart disease, hypertension, and depression. Recipes include the Long-Life Elixir, Male Toner Tea, and Fertility and Potency Syrup. Also includes a dosage chart and extensive profiles of the most useful herbs for enhancing men's health. 96 pages. Paperback. ISBN 1-58017-151-6.

Saw Palmetto for Men & Women, by David Winston. Respected herbalist Winston brings a new perspective to using this popular herb for both men's and women's health problems such as prostate enlargement, male baldness, ovarian pain and cysts, infertility, cystic acne, anorexia, and as a booster for the immune system. 128 pages. Paperback. ISBN 1-58017-206-7.

These books and other Storey Books are available at your bookstore, farm store, garden center, or directly from Storey Books, Schoolhouse Road, Pownal, Vermont 05261, or by calling 1-800-441-5700. Or visit our Web site at www.storey.com.